HON

THE BABY IN
THE PRODUCE
AISLE!

Alison Rhodes

Course Technology PTR
A part of Cengage Learning

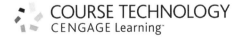

COURSE TECHNOLOGY
CENGAGE Learning™

Australia, Brazil, Japan, Korea, Mexico, Singapore, Spain, United Kingdom, United States

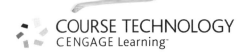

COURSE TECHNOLOGY
CENGAGE Learning

Honey, I Lost the Baby in the Produce Aisle!
Alison Rhodes

Publisher and General Manager, Course Technology PTR:
Stacy L. Hiquet

Associate Director of Marketing:
Sarah Panella

Manager of Editorial Services:
Heather Talbot

Marketing Manager:
Mark Hughes

Senior Acquisitions Editor:
Emi Smith

Project Editor and Copy Editor:
Marta Justak

Interior Layout:
Jill Flores

Cover Designer:
Luke Fletcher

Indexer:
Sharon Shock

Proofreader:
Sue Boshers

For product information and technology assistance, contact us at **Cengage Learning Customer & Sales Support, 1-800-354-9706**

For permission to use material from this text or product, submit all requests online at **cengage.com/permissions** Further permissions questions can be emailed to **permissionrequest@cengage.com**.

All trademarks are the property of their respective owners.

All images © Cengage Learning unless otherwise noted.

Library of Congress Control Number: 2011923927

ISBN-13: 978-1-4354-5970-0

ISBN-10: 1-4354-5970-9

Course Technology, a part of Cengage Learning
20 Channel Center Street
Boston, MA 02210
USA

Cengage Learning is a leading provider of customized learning solutions with office locations around the globe, including Singapore, the United Kingdom, Australia, Mexico, Brazil, and Japan. Locate your local office at: **international.cengage.com/region**.

Cengage Learning products are represented in Canada by Nelson Education, Ltd.

For your lifelong learning solutions, visit **courseptr.com**.

Visit our corporate Web site at **cengage.com**.

Printed in the United States of America
1 2 3 4 5 6 7 13 12 11

This book is dedicated to my little angel Connor who put me on the path I was meant to travel.

Acknowledgments

This book was truly a process of labor and love. It would never have been possible without the support, love, and encouragement of my entire "family."

It was important to me that I provide the most accurate, detailed, and professional advice I could on babyproofing and product installation. That would not have been possible without the tremendous input from Chris Benedict, "babyproofer extraordinaire" for Safety Mom Solutions, and one of the nicest men…and dads…I've ever met!

Everyone should have a Stephanie in their lives. Thank you to Stephanie Goodman who laughed with me, cried with me, and kicked me in the butt at exactly the right times! Her passion and belief in our mission at Safety Mom is what has led us to where we are today.

Thank you to my Mom. I only hope I can be as good a mother as you are. Your optimism and unconditional love for everyone is inspirational beyond words. I'm blessed having you in my life.

For my kids: Spencer, Kelsey, and Hannah and my wonderful step-kids: Emma and Wyatt, please see that you can do anything you set your mind to (even when you don't know what the heck you're doing!). Thank you for supporting Mommy and being my daily source of inspiration.

There aren't words to express my gratitude to my wonderful fiancé Greg Jacobson. His calm, steadfast, and abundant love has carried me through exhausting days and nights putting this book together.

About the Author

Alison Rhodes, The Safety Mom, has exploded onto the national scene as the preeminent voice on safety, wellness, and healthy living. From environmental toxins and healthy eating to sports injuries and cyber bullying, The Safety Mom is always on the lookout for the issues facing children—newborns to teens—as well as the entire family.

After experiencing the death of her child from SIDS, Alison became committed to saving children's lives. Over the years, Alison has expanded her career platform to include a gamut of vital issues facing families. As a mom of a special needs child, Alison has become a strong advocate for early intervention and programs that teach tolerance in our schools.

Alison believes that children's parents are their greatest safety advocates, and she coaches parents that when it comes to dealing with their children, it's important to be parents first and friends second. Her ability to connect with parents in a down-to-earth, uplifting, and engaging manner while providing important information has made Alison a popular guest on many national television shows including *The Today Show*, *Fox & Friends*, *Good Morning America*, *CNN International*, *CNBC Squawk Box*, and *The Doctors*.

Both her newsletter, *The Safety Scoop*, and blog, The Safety Chronicles, as well as regular articles on popular parenting sites such as Parenting Weekly and Baby Weekly, reach thousands of parents every month with tips and advice that help parents sort through the hype and get to the facts.

Alison resides in Connecticut with her three children.

Contents

Introduction xi

Chapter 1
Congratulations—You're Pregnant... OMG! 1
Cord Blood Banking—What Your Doctor Didn't Tell You 2
Understanding the Roles of Midwives and Doulas 4
Stillbirth and Counting Kicks 7
Newborn Screening Tests—Are They Worth It? 7

Chapter 2
Registering for the Shower—Must Haves 9
Do Your Homework First 10
A Word About Hand-Me-Downs 11
Cribs and Co-Sleepers 12
Car Seats/Travel Systems 13
    Infant Car Seats 14
    Travel System 15
    Convertible Seats 16
    Proper Positioning of a Car Seat 17
What About Taxis? 18
Play Yards 20
High Chairs 21
Bouncy Seats and Activity Centers 23
Bath Tubs 25

Chapter 3
Bringing Your Baby Home—Now What? 29
Do Dogs *Really* Eat Diapers? 30
There's Safety in Numbers...Not! 33
Spreading the Love, Not the Germs 35
A Word About SIDS 36
Postpartum Depression 39
What's Your Escape Plan? 40
Carbon Monoxide: The Silent Killer 42

Chapter 4
Babyproofing Do-It-Yourself 45
Gates 47
    Hardware-Mounted Gates 47
    Pressure-Mounted Walk-Through Gates 48

Pressure-Mounted Gates 49
Sectional Gates for Wide or Irregular Openings 49
Hearth Gates. 50
Retractable Gates 50
Wood Versus Metal Gates. 50
Installation How-To's 51
Windows 57
Installation How-To's 59
Window Blind Cords 61
Installation How-To's 62
Drawers/Cabinets Locks. 62
Installation How-To's 63
Doors 67
Installation How-To's 68
Electrical Cords 73
Furniture Strapping and Bracing 74
Installation How-To's 74

Chapter 5
Yes, They Will Try to Climb into the Toilet 77

Kitchen 79
Set Up a Safe Area in the Kitchen 79
Lock Down Appliances. 80
Installation How-To's 82
Cooking with Kids. 84
Bathrooms 86
Home Offices/Gyms/Media Rooms 88
Outdoor Areas. 90
Back-over Accidents 92
Play Areas 92
Pools and Hot Tubs 93

Chapter 6
Special Situations. 95

My Story 96
Autism 98
Symptoms of Autism 99
Potential Medical Problems and More Symptoms 100
Trust Yourself 101
That Feeling of Guilt 102
Get Support 102
Childproofing Is a Must 103
Cerebral Palsy 104

Contents

The Role of Environmental Toxins. 106
    Chemical Toxins 106
What to Do About Toxins 108
    Clear the Air 108
    Toss the Cleaners 108
You Are What You Eat 109
    Get the Lead Out 109

Chapter 7
Taking Baby Out—You Can't Babyproof the World 111

Going Outside 112
Riding Toy Safety 115
Surviving the Playground Jungle 117
    Interacting with Other Children. 118
    Checking Out Playground Equipment 118
Pools and Beaches 122
    Drowning Prevention 124
    Pool Drains 126
    Surf Warnings. 127
Amusement Parks 127
Play Date Do's and Don'ts 128
When the Play Date Is for You 131
Shopping Cart Injuries 131
Organized Sports and Activities 132

Chapter 8
Vacation Safety—A Map for Not Losing Your Mind 135

What You Need to Know Before Traveling Abroad 136
    Proper Documentation 136
    Packing 137
    Natural Disasters and Travel Warnings 138
Preparing for the Flight 139
Making It Through Airport Security 140
Seat, Restraints, and Regulations for the Plane. 141
    How to Secure the Seat. 143
    Changing Diapers on a Plane. 144
    Feeding Baby on a Plane. 145
Road Trips. 145
Making Grandma's House Safe. 147
Grandparents Babysitting 148
    Plan Ahead for the Unknown 148
    Cribs and High Chairs 149
    Pets and Plugs 150
    Pools and Hot Tubs. 151

Hotels and Resorts 152
    Kid Friendly 152
    Check for Bedbugs 152
    Orient Your Kids 153
    Potential Hazards 153
    Other Things to Consider. 154
Cruises 156
Theme Parks 156
Ski Vacations 159

Chapter 9
Getting Back into the World 161

The Great Divide. 162
No, Mary Poppins Does Not Exist—Finding the Next Best Thing. 163
Au Pairs 164
    State Department Guidelines 165
    Challenges of an Au Pair 166
Nannies 168
    The Costs of a Nanny. 169
    Nanny Checks. 169
    Be Clear About Your Expectations. 171
Day Care Centers 172
Family Day Care 176
Finding a Babysitter. 177

Chapter 10
Holidays, Seasonal, and Special Occasions 179

Christmas and Hanukkah 180
    Christmas Trees 182
    Menorahs 184
    Decorations. 184
    Party Patrol 184
    Holiday Baking 185
    Toys. 186
    Shopping Safety 187
    What to Do When Your Child Gets Lost at the Mall. 188
    Escalators 189
    Germs 190
Winter Safety. 190
    The Right Clothes Make a Difference 191
    Sports and Their Dangers 191
    Frost Nip and Frostbite 192
Summer Safety. 193
    Check Equipment. 193
    Beware of Trampolines 193

Contents

Grilling and Sunscreen 194

Drowning 194

Dehydration 195

The Dangers of Lyme Disease and Bee Stings. 195

Camping 198

Halloween Safety. 200

Birthday Parties 202

Party Details to Consider 202

Decorations and Balloons. 203

4th of July 204

Conclusion. 205

Appendices

Diaper Bag Checklist. 207

Nanny Questionnaire 209

Au Pair Questionnaire. 211

Index 213

Introduction

How many times have you thought, "I wish my baby came with a manual." We're thrust into the world of parenthood with very little preparation. And, as many veteran parents know, it's almost impossible to explain to the soon-to-be parent the extraordinary joys and anxieties that will be a part of the journey they are about to undertake.

What you need to know is that when you have kids, stuff happens. Every one of us deals with the guilty parent syndrome at some point—I forgot to close the baby gate at the top of the stairs, the car seat wasn't secured tightly enough, my toddler wandered out the patio door without my noticing, and countless other incidents. The reality is that we try to be the best parents we can be, but accidents do happen—we're only human.

And do you know what? It's OK! We need to stop comparing ourselves to the mom down the street. You know her, the one who seems to have it all together. Her house is spotlessly clean, her kids have never seen the inside of an emergency room, and she serves only organic, healthy treats. Yes, she may seem to be doing everything right, but I guarantee you that there's something that even she feels she can do better.

This book is not meant to lecture you on how to become the safest parent. As "The Safety Mom," I try to offer practical tips and advice. Some may be right for you, others might not. You are your child's best safety advocate. I'm here simply to offer some options, a menu, if you will, for you to peruse to find some solutions to your specific challenges and offer insight on other situations you might not have previously considered.

There's also the theory that our kids need to explore and get some scrapes and bruises so that they learn about dangers on their own, somewhat akin to *The Blessing of a Skinned Knee*'s philosophy. I don't necessarily disagree with this. We can't keep our kids in hermetically sealed bubbles all their lives. They will be out and about visiting friends' and relatives' homes that are minefields for curious toddlers. So, for those of you who thought this book might present every safety hazard imaginable and prey on the neuroses of hyper-vigilant parents, fear not. We can't live in paranoia. We can only take realistic precautions, be aware of potential hazards, and do our best.

This book is about those first years. It begins even before you bring your baby home from the hospital for the first time.

These are the real "war stories" and the safety and wellness tips that others just don't tell you!

Chapter 1

Congratulations— You're Pregnant… OMG!

I remember when I first realized I was pregnant—it was an amazing feeling of disbelief coupled with indescribable joy. Then the panic set in. What the heck did I know about being a mother? Me, the person who swore she'd never drive a minivan, couldn't imagine cleaning up puke, and had no idea how you're supposed to potty train, was now going to be responsible for a little baby's well-being! Whether your plans include having a baby or it was a "surprise," as soon as that little stick turns blue, your life changes, and no one can prepare you for the rollercoaster ride that it will become. Sure, well-meaning friends and relatives will give you their war stories and offer plenty of advice, regardless of your desire to hear it, but this is fairly generic information. Here are some things that you might not have heard about and might never be told.

The Things We Do for Love

You Can't Make This Up

When my husband and I were having difficulties getting pregnant, we decided to do in-vitro fertilization. Because the doctor wanted as fresh a "sample" as possible, he needed my husband to "provide one" at the office. He sent my husband into a public bathroom...let me stress...A PUBLIC BATHROOM at the medical building to "get it done." My husband was, needless to say, less than thrilled to have to do this in a public restroom but there was no choice. Things weren't proceeding as quickly as possible and before it "could happen" the lights went out in the bathroom, and he was left standing in pitch darkness in the stall. Since he was in a "compromised" state, he wasn't sure what to do but was worried someone would come in and find out what was happening. It turns out that the lights in the bathroom were on motion sensors and would turn off if there were no motion for 60 seconds! When my husband went back in to explain the dilemma to the doctor, he told my husband that it still needed to be done if we wanted to perform the procedure. When he asked the doctor if he knew how to disengage the sensor in the restroom, the doctor calmly replied, "I have no idea, I never go in there. I only use my private restroom here in the office!"

Patty Riley, Tampa, FL

Cord Blood Banking—What Your Doctor Didn't Tell You

One topic that is often overlooked is that of cord blood banking and the potential life-saving benefits associated with it. Cord blood banking is the process of collecting and storing the blood that remains in your baby's umbilical cord after it has been cut. This blood, similar to bone marrow, is a rich source of unique stem cells that can be used in the treatment of numerous medical issues your child might face, including cancer, cerebral palsy, juvenile diabetes, and brain injury. While you may find brochures in your OB/GYNs office about cord blood banking, unfortunately, many doctors don't discuss this option with their patients as a matter of course. Patients are sometimes led to believe that, unless there is family history of a disease, there is no need to store their baby's blood. This is a case in which parents are not being given sufficient information to make the best decision for their family. Every day, doctors and researchers are finding new benefits for saving cord blood stem cells. There is tremendous anecdotal evidence of how cord blood has saved or improved thousands of children's lives. This is especially true with premature infants.

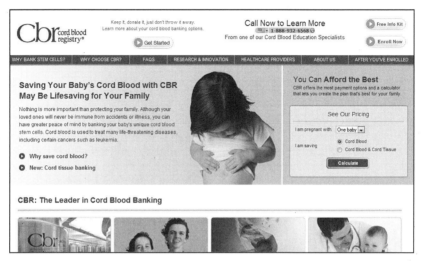

Here is one cord blood banking site.

Two years ago, one of my friends delivered her twins at just 28 weeks. When I learned she was in the hospital and about to deliver, I immediately reached out to her to be sure she had planned to store the babies' cord blood. Needless to say, she and her husband were scared and overwhelmed. They barely heard what I was saying and understood even less. But I was determined to make them listen. The first comment from the expectant dad was, "Why didn't we hear about this from our doctor?" Good question. Why *aren't* parents given more information about this process? But at that moment, I didn't have time to argue with him or explain it. I needed to get him to understand that this could potentially save his children's lives. Fortunately, my persistence paid off, and I convinced them of the importance of storing their babies' blood. We were able to get a kit delivered by a Cord Blood Registry representative as she was being wheeled into the delivery room. I'm happy to report that both boys are now happy and healthy toddlers, but their cord blood is still available if they ever need it.

Cord blood banking is insurance for the future. While it's something that one hopes never to use, it has the potential to save lives. It's important to do your own research to understand the benefits and then talk to your OB/GYN.

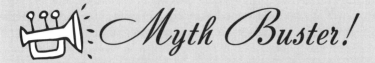

Myth Buster!

Cord Blood Benefits

Myth: If there is no family history of a genetic disease there is no reason to bank your child's cord blood.

Every day the uses of cord blood and the diseases it can help treat are increasing. Clinical trials are now underway for the use of cord blood stems cells in the treatment of traumatic brain injury. Cord blood is also being researched for use in regenerative medicine to treat cerebral palsy and juvenile diabetes. Nearly 80 serious diseases have been treated with cord blood stem cells, including sickle cell disease, Tay-Sachs disease, non-Hodgkin's lymphoma, and brain tumors. Banking your child's cord blood is insurance for the future.

There are both private and public banking options for your child's cord blood. If you decide that you wish to store your child's cord blood for potential use in the future, you can contact one of the private banks. It's not necessary for the storage facility to be located near you, but rather be sure it's one that is well established. If you decide that you don't want to store your child's blood, you can donate it to a public bank. Public banks store cord blood anonymously and can be used by people in need of transplants and those with leukemia and immune disorders. But, because it's not the patient's own cord blood, there's no guarantee that it will be able to be used.

I've run across so many parents whose child has ultimately become sick, and they regret not having stored her blood. This is something to seriously be researched and considered when you're pregnant.

Understanding the Roles of Midwives and Doulas

When I was pregnant with my first son, I decided that I wanted to have a completely natural birth—no drugs, a non-hospital environment, a midwife, and delivery in a bathtub. My mother thought I was crazy and chalked it up to my time spent living in Los Angeles. When she was pregnant with me back in the 1960s, they drugged her up and when she awoke, she had a baby in her arms, which, in her mind, was a much easier process. While I agree that 15 years ago natural births without drugs were a little uncommon, women were beginning to think that it was worth a try. Men were starting to bestow non-epidural gifts on their wives as an incentive. Oh, how I wish I could get a genie to grant me just *one* wish and have men experience childbirth!

I was fortunate that one of my best friend's aunts was a midwife in the town nearby. She practiced at the birth cottages that were associated with the local hospital. On my first visit to the cottages, I knew immediately that this was the right choice for my labor and delivery. The "cottage" featured five rooms, each one decorated like a quaint bedroom at a bed and breakfast. Monitors and other medical equipment were discreetly hidden in closets. Even better were the bathrooms with the giant sauna tubs where I could labor. I had read that laboring in water not only eased the pain for the mother, but was also a much less traumatic delivery experience for the baby.

For those of you who are unfamiliar with midwives, this is certainly something to consider. A midwife is a person who works with the mom-to-be and the entire family to offer guidance and support throughout the pregnancy, labor, and delivery. Unlike a traditional OB/GYN, a midwife focuses on the entire family and encourages everyone to become involved. They listen to the mother's personal preferences, as well as the cultural considerations of moms-to-be. They allow a woman to be more in control of her birthing process and help to reduce the need for invasive procedures and medication. What I didn't realize initially is that, for lengthy labors that are progressing normally it is impossible for nurses to be with you constantly. Certainly, for the first time around it was comforting for me to have my midwife. During labor in a hospital setting with an OB/GYN, for a majority of the time, your sole source of company might be a sleepy partner and TV reruns. A midwife is constantly present, offering you support and monitoring you. Additionally, you won't have a prior relationship with the nurse who is monitoring you during delivery. On the other hand, by the time you're in labor, you will have established a close relationship with your midwife who will better understand your needs at that time. A midwife can offer the calm, assuring coaching that a nurse won't and your spouse absolutely can't. She can suggest trying different positions to help ease labor pains and offer help to make your labor progress more rapidly. And while she will coach you and encourage you to avoid the use of pain medication and other interventions, if your labor stalls or the baby is in distress, she will support you in your choice for Pitocin, which will increase contractions, or the need for a C-section.

The use of midwives is increasing steadily. In fact, over the past 20 years, the number of women who have chosen to use a midwife has doubled. There's good reason for this. According to the latest research, women with low-risk pregnancies who utilize a midwife receive fewer episiotomies, are more successful with vaginal births after a C-section (VBAC), reduce the use of forceps, and require less pain medication. And the rate of C-sections is lower. Women with midwives ended up with a C-section only 13 percent of the time, in contrast to the national average of 21 percent.

While a midwife can prescribe medicine, she will work with a physician should any medical complications arise during your pregnancy or labor and delivery. But your regular pre-natal visits will be with the midwife. Midwives can practice in hospitals, but in many places, free-standing birthing centers or similar facilities are located near hospitals. These birthing centers offer families the benefit of delivering their baby in a non-hospital setting, while still providing the capability to move to the hospital if a medical emergency or the need for an emergency C-section arises.

There are different accreditations for midwives, and it's important to understand the distinctions to find one that's right for you. The American College of Nurse-Midwives (ACNM) offers two accreditations—a Certified Nurse-Midwife and a Certified Midwife. A Certified Nurse-Midwife holds a nursing degree and has an RN license, as well as certification as a midwife. She is able to write prescriptions, order epidurals, and manage the administration of Pitocin. At times, she may also assist in a C-section if required. This is the only certification accepted by the American College of Obstetricians and Gynecology (ACOG) and most CNMs (Certified Nurse Midwives) practice in hospitals or free-standing birth centers associated with hospitals.

A Certified Midwife (CM) is not required to have a degree in nursing but must pass the same certification exam as that required of CNMs. While they are not recognized by ACOG, they generally have the same status as CNMs in most states, although state guidelines can be confusing. The other major organization is the Midwives Alliance of North America (MANA), which offers midwives accreditation as Certified Professional Midwives (CPMs). Their training includes schooling and an apprenticeship and requires the passing of an exam. Certificates between the two organizations are not interchangeable and standards for CMs and CNMs are more stringent. To find a midwife, visit the ACNM's Web site at *www.acnm.org* and the MANA Web site at *www.mana.org*.

With my last daughter, I unfortunately no longer had access to my midwife. So, while I selected an OB/GYN for my medical care, I also hired a doula to help care for me. The doula was amazing! My labor was quite long, and she stayed by my side the entire time. My then husband actually fell asleep, and my doula worked with me to try different positions, massaged my back, and just helped me relax. Similar to a midwife, a doula will help guide and coach a woman through labor and delivery. She'll help the woman's partner be as involved as he or she wants to be and will work with the mom with different positions to ease the pain, coach her through contractions, and provide massages and other strategies to make the labor process easier. After delivery, a doula will coach the new mom in initiating and successfully establishing breastfeeding. As with midwives, studies have shown that when a doula is involved in a birth, there are fewer complications and shorter labors, less use of pain medication, and a reduction in the need for Pitocin, the use of forceps, and the need for a C-section. To learn more about doulas or to find one in your area, visit DONA International at *www.dona.org*.

Stillbirth and Counting Kicks

While miscarriage and stillbirth are things no expectant mom wants to think about, unfortunately they are a sad reality for many women. I will admit that when I was pregnant I skipped over the section in the pregnancy books about SIDS because I never dreamed it would happen to me (or I just didn't want to think about it, I'm not sure which), but sadly it did.

DID YOU KNOW?   DID YOU KNOW?   DID YOU KNOW?   DID YOU KNOW?

Rate of Stillbirth

While stillbirth rates have declined by almost 50 percent in the last 30 years, 25,000 stillbirths still occur every year.

DID YOU KNOW? DID YOU KNOW? DID YOU KNOW? DID YOU KNOW?

Stillbirth is considered any fetal demise in utero of a fetus older than 20 weeks gestation. There can be a variety of causes for a stillbirth, including problems with the placenta, birth defects, lack of oxygen, infections, maternal high blood pressure or diabetes, and umbilical cord accidents.

In many cases, there is nothing a woman can do to prevent stillbirth, but good prenatal care is important, as well as closely monitoring your baby's kicking for any irregularities. By performing a kick count at the same time every day during your last trimester, you can also help your doctor monitor your baby's health. Doctors recommend that parents start counting and keeping track of their baby's kicks beginning with the 28th week of pregnancy (earlier for high-risk pregnancies). By doing kick counting daily, you will get to know your baby's normal movement pattern within a week or two. By using a kick count chart, you and your doctor will be able to tell if there are any changes in your baby's normal pattern. Studies show that a major decrease in your baby's normal amount of movement could be a signal that there's a problem.

Newborn Screening Tests—Are They Worth It?

When I was pregnant with my second child, I began researching and asking questions about newborn screening tests. I wasn't really informed of the additional testing that could be requested when I was pregnant with my first son, and while this screening would not have saved his life, these tests can definitely detect rare disorders that might otherwise go unnoticed until too late.

Every newborn is screened within the first few days of life for potentially fatal disorders that are not always apparent at birth. Many of these are metabolic disorders (often called "inborn errors of metabolism") that interfere with the body's use of nutrients to maintain healthy tissues and produce energy. Other disorders that screenings can detect include problems with hormones or the blood. In general, metabolic and other inherited disorders can hinder an infant's normal physical and mental development in a variety of ways. And parents can pass along the gene for a certain disorder without even knowing that they are carriers.

Many states use the tandem mass spectrometry (or MS/MS), which can screen for more than 20 inherited metabolic disorders with a single drop of blood. All states and U.S. territories screen newborns for phenylketonuria (PKU), hypothyroidism, galactosemia, and sickle cell disease. Unfortunately, there is no federal mandate or standard for newborn screening, so each state operates its own program. In some states, including Maryland and Wyoming, testing is not mandatory. And the number and types of conditions for which each state tests varies greatly, so you should check not only with your OB/GYN, but also with the hospital where you plan to deliver to see which tests they offer. Some hospitals go beyond the state requirements and do additional testing. Almost all states test for at least 30 disorders, but it's possible to test for more than 50. You can visit the National Newborn Screening & Genetics Resource Center Web site at *http://genes-r-us.uthscsa.edu/parentpage.htm* to determine which disorders a particular state tests for and a list of commercial labs that will do additional testing for a fee.

Most, but not all, states also require newborns to have a hearing test before they're discharged from the hospital. It's critical that a baby's hearing be checked within the first three weeks of life. A hearing problem can interfere with the development of early speech and language skills, but if caught and treated, could prevent problems from developing later.

According to the March of Dimes and The American Academy of Pediatrics, you should consider additional testing if you meet the following conditions:

* You have a family history of an inherited disorder.
* You have previously given birth to a child who is affected by a disorder.
* You have an infant in your family who has died because of a suspected metabolic disorder.

Unfortunately, some of the metabolic disorders that can be detected have no cure, so parents may feel they would prefer not to know. But science and medicine are making new advances every day and understanding your child's physical issues will allow you to seek help in the future.

All of these concerns—and your baby hasn't even been born yet. While it might seem daunting, the old saying "an ounce of prevention" is completely true.

Chapter 2

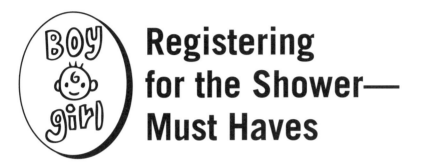 **Registering
for the Shower—
Must Haves**

I'll never forget the first time I was pregnant and walked into a baby store. I had no idea what I really needed or how much "stuff" was out there for babies. I looked like a pregnant deer caught in the headlights. What I discovered after spending a great deal of money is that half of the products aren't even necessary. Every year, new products come onto the market aimed at making the lives of moms and dads easier. Some of it is great, and some of it just pure hype. There are a few products that fall into the "must-have" category and others that are definitely just "nice to have." The problem is you never really know what your baby will actually use. Sure, your sister's baby might have adored his swing and fallen asleep every time he was placed in it, but your baby might hate it. The best bet is to buy the basics first—a crib, car seat or travel system, a high chair, a bathtub, a play yard, and some type of activity seat.

Do Your Homework First

Once you've decided what to buy, the question becomes which brand, model, and design. There are endless products on the market, but how do you know which makes the most sense for you and which is safe? Due to all the recalls that have been issued over the past few years, it's become quite confusing. In fact, an analysis of recalls conducted by the Consumer Products Safety Commission shows that more than 40 nursery products involving more than 21 million units were recalled in 2009.

Prior to registering for something at a "big box" baby products store (or even a smaller boutique), do your homework. It's one thing to read about a product in a baby magazine, but nothing can compare to asking a few moms who already own the item what they think of it. If something is difficult to clean, hard to put up or take down, or cumbersome to use, you want to know about that ahead of time. You will find that, once you join the "sisterhood of mothers," your best source of info on any product will come from other moms who've test driven it. Of course, it's also important to read reviews and gather data from trusted organizations.

Two great sources of information on product safety are the Consumer Product Safety Commission (CPSC) at *www.cpsc.gov* and the Juvenile Products Manufacturers Association (JPMA) at *www.jpma.org*. The CPSC offers parents the ability to sign up to receive emails about baby products that have been recalled. On a monthly basis, there are numerous recalls on products, which is why it's so important not only to mail in your warranty and registration cards, but also to keep a list of all of the specifics of each product, including year and model number.

The JPMA is a national trade organization comprised of more than 300 manufacturers of juvenile products. Members must submit their products to be tested by an independent facility and meet the guidelines set by safety standards developer, ASTM International. If their products pass, manufacturers are able to place the JPMA's Safety Certification Seal on them, which lets consumers know that this product meets certain safety standards. The JPMA has a great area on its site for parents to learn more about the program, find products that have been certified, and get additional parenting information.

You Can't Make This Up

My Beautiful Two-for-One Gifts

When I was pregnant with my twins, I didn't have much experience with babies so the day I went to do my baby registry I was more than a little confused. I was browsing through the shelves and overheard another woman talking to a friend, holding up a package, and asking how many "onesies" she should buy. After she left, I went over to look at them since I had never heard of onesies. I figured this was specifically for women who were having one child so I went up to the sales clerk asked where I could find the "twosies."

Jillian Phillips, Phoenix, AZ

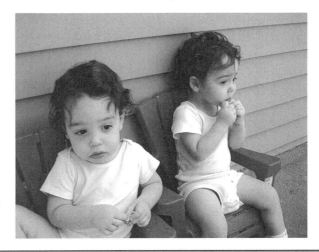

Two boys in two onesies—no twosies for sale.

A Word About Hand-Me-Downs

Let's face it—babies are expensive! Parents are always trying to find ways to save money, but you should be careful when it comes to used baby furniture and products. There is often the possibility that something has been recalled, and the previous owner may not even be aware of it. And safety standards continually change. Slats on a crib, for example, should be no more than 2 3/8" apart to prevent strangulation. In 2010, we saw the recall of millions of drop-side cribs due to concerns regarding entrapment and strangulation. Screws may be missing and parts could be broken on used baby furniture or products. Car seats, in particular, should never be bought secondhand. You have no way of knowing if it has been involved in a car accident and compromised in some way.

Check out any product that you receive at the Consumer Products Safety Commission Web site to see if it has been recalled. The site has a feature that allows consumers to sign up and receive email alerts regarding the recall of any infant or child product. You can also check to see if any product you receive as a gift or have used in the past has been recalled. Even products that have received the JPMA seal may still have been recalled; in many instances, this is due to products being assembled improperly or for other issues not related to the testing method.

Cribs and Co-Sleepers

Clearly, one of the most important baby products is a crib. Not only is this where your little one will be spending a great deal of time, but it is usually the focal point of the nursery. The question is one of safety: what crib is the safest and most secure for your baby? Toward the end of 2009, we saw the first recall of millions of drop-side cribs. These are cribs in which one or two of the sides drops down, making it easier to reach in and pick up or lay down your baby. The reason these cribs were recalled was due to broken and missing parts, faulty design, and assembly issues—namely, parents not following the manufacturers' instructions on how to put these cribs together properly. As a result, several strangulation and suffocation deaths occurred when babies became trapped between the mattress and the side of the crib, and the babies were strangled or suffocated. Manufacturing of drop-side cribs was banned in the summer of 2010, but unfortunately, thousands of these cribs will still be on the market for some time. And many parents believe that, since their first child was safe in a drop-side crib, the subsequent child will be safe as well, or that it's okay to give the crib to someone else as a hand-me-down.

Drop-side cribs should not be used under any circumstances! But a crib with fixed sides is still the safest place for a baby. While we have heard a great deal about the statistics of babies dying due to issues with drop-side cribs, what we've heard less about is the number of deaths caused by babies sleeping in adult sleeping areas. There's a great deal of heated debate about co-sleeping with your baby. Some people vehemently support the "family bed," but the American Academy of Pediatrics and other organizations strongly advise against co-sleeping because of the risk of suffocation and other dangers. But let's face it, we need our sleep and it's so convenient to bring your baby into the bed when you're nursing or if your baby is fussy. There are other alternatives, however, that offer a compromise. An infant co-sleeper that attaches to the side of your bed will allow you to have the baby right next to you, but in her own sleeping environment. There are several manufacturers of co-sleepers, but one of the original ones is the Arm's Reach co-sleeper. I loved this one and used it with all of my kids. Sleeping areas that are not safe for your baby include water beds, futons, sofas, and other adult sleeping areas.

Keep in mind that all those beautiful comforters and crib bumpers that are displayed are not safe to have in the crib. A crib should have a firm, tight-fitting mattress with a snug-fitting sheet. Never place pillows, blankets, or stuffed animals in a crib, as these are all SIDS risks. Soft, fluffy bumpers are not only a danger in terms of SIDS, but can also be used as leverage to climb out of the crib once your baby gets older. Parents worry that in the winter months their baby will be cold without a blanket in the crib. There are several great products on the market that will keep a baby warm yet pose no hazard. Two of my top picks are the Snooze Wrap and the Snooze Sack. The Snooze Wrap allows for easy swaddling and provides head support and tummy comfort for the baby. It attaches directly to the mattress so you never have to worry about your baby rolling over or getting too near the edge of the crib. Once your baby grows out of the Snooze Wrap, the Snooze Sack is a great option for keeping your baby warm and safe without a traditional blanket. Both of these can be found at most retailers and by visiting the company's Web site at *www.soothetime.com*.

Car Seats/Travel Systems

One of the most important purchases is a car seat or travel system for your baby. There are a myriad of different designs and styles from which to choose, but first-time parents often have no clue what they need. It would certainly be much easier if every car seat and car was created equal, but that just isn't the case.

Car accidents are the leading cause of death for children ages 1 to 14 years of age. Selecting the right car seat is vital in helping keep your baby safe. When considering which car seat to purchase, it's important that you consult your car manual, as well as the car seat instruction booklet to make sure it is compatible with your vehicle. Cars manufactured after 2002 have the LATCH (Lower Anchors and Tethers for Children) system. LATCH consists of lower attachments on child seats and a set of tether anchors in the vehicle to hold the child seat in place without the use of the vehicle's seat belts. All car seats will ultimately have the LATCH system, but if your car is older than 2002, you will still be able to use the car seat. There are many great car seats on the market, but be sure the one you've selected also has been side-impact tested. The National Highway Traffic Safety Administration has developed an "ease-of-use" five-star rating program to help parents determine the right car seat for their particular needs and car.

Types of car seats include: an infant seat, convertible car seat, and a travel system. Each has its pros and cons.

Infant Car Seats

Infant car seats are only used for the first few months of your baby's life, or the first year at most. An infant car seat will only accommodate a baby up to 12 months of age and 20 pounds. Check the manufacturer's guidelines for your particular seat because some of them will only hold a baby up to 15 pounds. While you will be spending more money buying another car seat once your baby grows out of an infant seat, the benefit of this seat is that it can be completely removed from the car and has a swing-up handle.

I can't imagine having to wake up a baby who's contentedly napping to remove her from a car seat. This is a great convenience when you're grocery shopping, heading out to the park, or just traveling to grandma's house. These seats come with a base that attaches into the car into which the seat snaps. It's a good idea to purchase an additional base for a second car or a caregiver who might be transporting your baby frequently. Don't try to secure an infant car seat without the base because it will not be properly positioned, and you run the risk of your baby's head falling forward and her airway becoming obstructed.

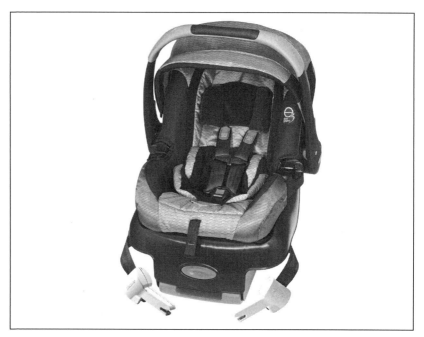

Evenflo makes this Secure System infant car seat.

Travel System

The travel system expands on the infant car seat and includes a stroller into which the infant seat will snap. Once your baby outgrows the infant car seat, most travel systems will convert into a stroller for your baby to sit in. Before purchasing one, really "test-drive" all the options. Ideally, you want to find one that you can steer with one hand and can fold down with a one-handed operation. A large basket underneath is also a plus. A few safety tips regarding strollers include the following:

* Never hang bags or other heavy objects from the handle because they can cause the entire stroller to fall backward with your child in it. I've witnessed this far too many times!

* When you're not pushing your stroller, be sure to engage the brake.

* Be careful placing hot liquids in the cup holder. If you hit a bump or trip, they can spill onto your baby causing a bad burn.

* Never allow an older child to stand on the back of the stroller. This, too, can cause it to tip over.

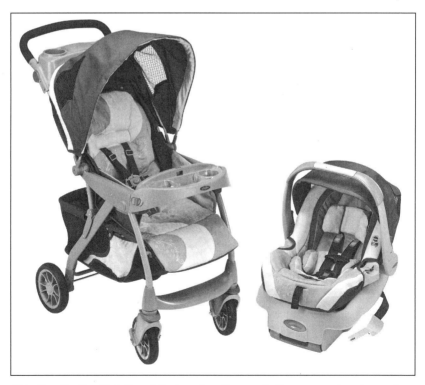

This Evenflo EuroTrek Travel System functions as both a car seat and a carrier.

Convertible Seats

A convertible seat is the only car seat you'll ever need. Most seats now hold babies from 5 to 80 and even 100 pounds. These seats start out as a rear-facing seat for infants and are then turned around for older children. Many of them have different recliner settings, and once they're installed, they don't need to be adjusted. But, unlike the infant seat, you won't be able to remove this from the car so you'll need to wake up a sleeping baby once you've arrived at your destination. Also, they tend to be heavy and cumbersome, so moving this seat between cars is not convenient.

Car seat models have different options, but be sure that whichever model you choose, it has been side-impact tested. More than 65 percent of car crashes involve some side-impact component. Be sure to read objective reviews online. While some car seats appear to be the best on the market, they might be quite difficult to install.

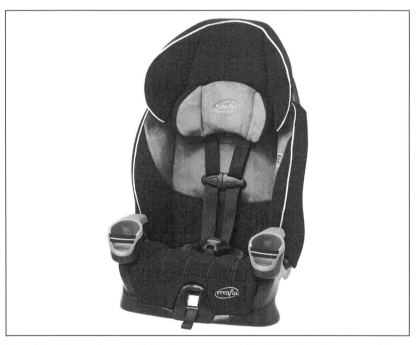

Evenflo's Maestro is a combination car seat with a five point harness and is convertible to a booster seat.

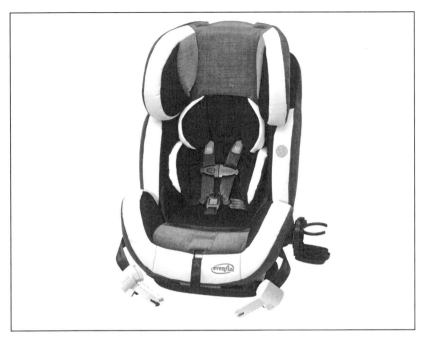

Evenflo's Symphony is also a combination car seat.

Proper Positioning of a Car Seat

Regardless of which type of car seat you choose, proper positioning and installation is critical. According to the National Highway Traffic Safety Administration, nearly 80 percent of car seats are installed or used improperly. And according to the Centers for Disease Control and Prevention, "among children under age 5, in 2006, an estimated 425 lives were saved by car and booster seat use." Here are some straightforward tips for keeping babies and children safe in car seats:

* Convertible car seats usually have a guide system on the side, which will clearly show if the seat is in the proper position. Be sure that you check this when installing the seat.

* Most towns have a police officer or firefighter who is certified in car seat installation. Many areas also offer car seat installation clinics. Before bringing your baby home from the hospital, check with one of these professionals to be sure you've installed your seat properly.

* Test a car seat before you purchase it to be sure it's easy for you to use. If you struggle with it, it's more likely that you will install it improperly at some point.

* Be sure your baby is secured into the car seat safely. With a five-point harness system, the shoulder clip should be at the level of the child's armpit. The straps need to be snug enough to hold the baby properly. No more than one small pinky finger should be able to fit between the baby and the strap at the shoulder.

* For rear-facing seats, the belt should be at or below the child's shoulders; for forward-facing seats, it should be at or above the child's shoulders.

* Keep in mind that children need to remain rear facing until they are 20 pounds and at least one year of age. Many pediatricians and experts suggest that babies stay in rear-facing seats up to two years of age.

* Remove your baby's heavy winter coat before strapping her in. Leaving it on will compromise the fit and security of the belt.

* Affix a baby mirror so you can easily see your baby while you're driving.

* Keep blankets out of reach from a sibling who could innocently put it over the head of a sleeping infant.

* If your car doesn't come equipped with built-in window shades, install one securely on the back window or windows.

* Most importantly, never leave your child unattended in a car even for a moment! On a 70-degree day, even with car windows slightly open, the temperature inside a car can exceed 120 degrees in 20 minutes and 150 degrees in 40 minutes.

* Place a neon-colored sticker on the side of the car seat with your child's vital statistics, including allergies to medicine and blood type, as well as an emergency contact number. If you're involved in a crash and rendered unconscious, emergency personnel will have a better idea of how to treat your child.

What About Taxis?

Having never lived with children in a metropolitan area, I always wondered what my New York City friends did when traveling. (Actually they've told me that what made most of them move out of the city wasn't the baby, but how much stuff went along *with* the baby.) You don't often see parents lugging around car seats, and I can't even imagine how difficult it would be with twins or bigger sets of multiples! Logic would dictate that if babies must ride in car seats in regular cars, there must be a law for cabs. Wrong! Review what the New York City Taxi and Limousine Commission Web site says in the Note.

Note

Car Seat Regulations for Taxis

Drivers of yellow medallion taxicabs and for-hire vehicles and their passengers, are exempt from laws regarding car seats and seatbelts. Keep in mind, the TLC encourages everyone in the vehicle to buckle his or her seatbelts while riding in a cab. There are no Taxi and Limousine Commission rules regarding this, as it is a State exemption. Passengers with children are encouraged to bring their own car seats, which the drivers must allow passengers to install.

***Note:** Children under the age of seven are permitted to sit on an adult's lap.*

A child under the age of seven sitting on a lap? That could be a 60-pound kid! And just what are you supposed to do, strap them in on top of you? Let's review a few laws of physics. (For those of you who missed that class in school like I did, I'll keep it easy.) In a crash, an unrestrained object has the force of its own weight multiplied by the speed of a crash. So, even a 40-pound child involved in a crash in which the car is traveling at only 20 miles per hour is going to hit the partition with 800 pounds of force. And, if you have a child strapped in with you or you're carrying your child in a front carrier, you will hit her with more than 1,000 pounds of force.

DID YOU KNOW? DID YOU KNOW? DID YOU KNOW? DID YOU KNOW?

Accidents in Taxis

Accidents in cabs *can* and *do* happen. According to a study conducted by Schaller Consulting, in 2004 there were 9,128 taxi and livery crashes in New York City that resulted in injuries and fatalities. Most alarming is the fact that passengers in taxi and livery cabs have almost doubled the chance of being seriously injured or killed than passengers in other vehicles. In fact, 21 percent of taxi passengers who were injured in a crash were seriously injured or killed. This is due primarily to passengers hitting the partition separating themselves and the driver, as well as the fact that many passengers still don't wear seat belts in cabs. So, when you're in a cab, buckle up and regardless of the rules, always have your child properly restrained in a car seat.

Play Yards

Without a doubt, the best purchase I made when my children were babies was my play yard. Play yards are not only a convenience for moms during the day, but they're a great sleeping area for your baby when you're on vacation or visiting friends or relatives. I remember when my kids were babies, I couldn't imagine having to run up and down stairs for nap times and diaper changes. This really is a terrific alternative for those times. There are several different designs of play yards for every budget and need. They can include a removable bassinet, a changing station, and music and lights. I find the ones with wheels are really convenient for moving around the house. When traveling with your baby, you'll find that they sleep better when they are in familiar surroundings. Not only does a play yard provide this, but also you don't have to worry whether the hotel has a safe crib or play yard. If you're going to be doing a great deal of traveling, look for one that's lightweight. If your baby will be spending frequent time at grandma's or a babysitter's house, it's a good idea to consider purchasing an additional play yard to be stored at the secondary location. If the play yard you purchase has a cradle, make sure it is sturdy and doesn't cradle your baby too tightly.

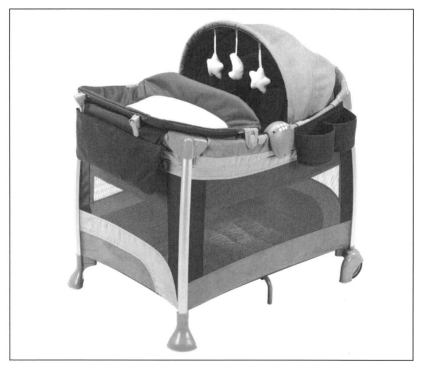

The Evenflo BabySuite Select play yard fills multiple purposes—for play and for napping.

A few things to keep in mind about play yards:

* As with a crib, you should never place pillows, comforters, or soft blankets in a play yard.

* Be sure that the play yard has been assembled properly and the legs are in the locked position.

* Consider the placement of the play yard. Move it away from lamp electrical cords or monitors or windows with window blind cords. Lamps can accidentally be pulled into the play yard, and the cords pose a strangulation hazard.

* If your child is napping in a play yard, be sure she is on her back.

High Chairs

While you might not be using it immediately, your baby's high chair is going to become an important household accessory. Whether she's snoozing in it or throwing food at you, your toddler will reach many milestones while strapped into her seat. High chairs have changed a great deal over the years, and thankfully, they have become safer. I almost had a knock-down fight with my mother who wanted to use an old-fashioned wooden hand-me-down high chair that she had received from a friend. The thing looked so unstable and dangerous, I wanted to scream. But, even while many of them are better today, recalls and accidents still occur. According to the Consumer Product Safety Commission, there were approximately 9,600 injuries due to high chair accidents in 1997, with falls being the primary cause.

Some safety tips for high chair use include the following:

* Always make sure chairs are properly assembled. Loose nuts and bolts or caps on the feet of the high chair that can be pulled off can pose a choking hazard.

* The chair should have both crotch and waist straps. Always use the crotch strap because your baby could slide underneath the waist strap.

* If your high chair has wheels, be sure that you always put on the brakes and engage the locking mechanism for a folding chair so it doesn't accidentally fold when your baby is in it.

* Never leave your child unattended in a high chair.

There are several types of high chairs from which to choose. My particular favorites are convertible or combination high chairs, which start out as a high chair and can then transform into a booster seat and activity desk as the child gets older. Some chairs can actually accommodate two children at once, as both a high chair and a booster seat.

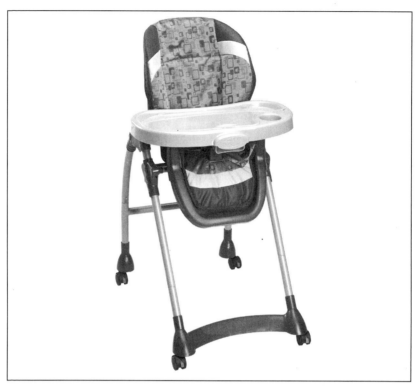

A booster high chair (this one by Summer Infants) makes eating easier.

Hook-on chairs that attach directly to the table are another option for older babies. These should never be used with infants or babies who are not able to support themselves. Hook-on chairs are great space savers and can be used on the go as well, but there are a few things to keep in mind.

* Follow the manufacturer's instructions carefully to be sure you are assembling it properly and following the weight guidelines.

* Check that the chair has strong clamps that are properly secured to the table. Never use on a glass table, single pedestal, leaf top, or one with a loose table top.

* Always attach it directly to the table, never to a tablecloth or placemat.

Bouncy Seats and Activity Centers

When you find out that you're pregnant, your doctor should hand you a dictionary of new words you'll need to learn. Bouncy seat, ExerSaucer, and Boppy (the brand name for the pillow that goes around a mother's stomach while she's nursing) are just a few of the words that were completely foreign to me before I had kids.

One of the most important items to have is a bouncy seat or activity center for your baby, but you'll most likely need both. Both are great places to keep your baby safe and have fun while you're busy doing something else or just need a few moments to yourself.

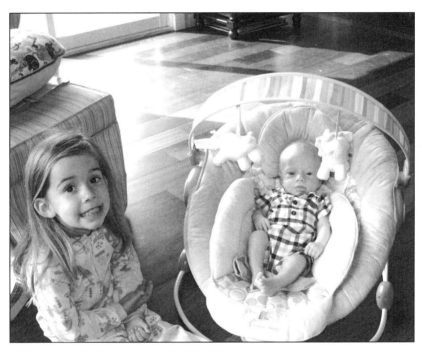

A bouncy seat lets everyone enjoy the baby.

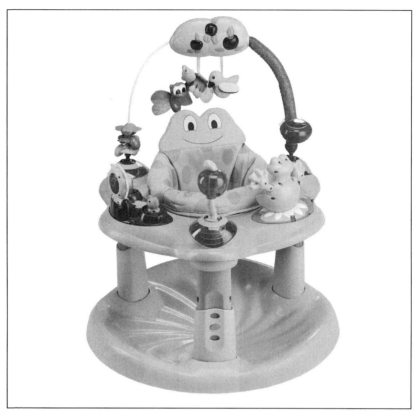

Evenflo ExerSaucer Jump & Learn Active Learning Center is a feast for baby's eyes.

If you haven't had a chance to research these items yet or are still in the clueless phase, bouncy seats are, quite literally, a seat that your child can be strapped into that bounces. They are terrific for soothing a fussy baby, and they usually come with a bar with dangling toys to keep him entertained. Here are a few safety precautions to follow with bouncy seats:

* Be sure that you always strap your baby in and never leave him unattended.

* Never place towels or blankets in the bouncy to prop your baby's head or to keep him warm, because they can become a suffocation hazard.

* Read the manufacturer's weight restrictions and other guidelines. Usually, it's between 18–30 pounds. A baby who is heavier could cause it to tip over. Some bouncy seats are also not manufactured to be used once a baby can sit up by himself.

✳ Never place the bouncy seat on a high surface, such as a table or countertop, because when he's in it, there's the possibility that he might wriggle out, or it could move and fall off.

✳ Keep the bouncy seat off soft surfaces, such as a bed, because if it tips over it can cause a suffocation hazard.

✳ Never carry the bouncy seat with your baby in it or by the toy handle.

My kids loved their activity center, and it was probably the best investment I ever made. These centers are stationary units that a baby can be placed in, and it essentially allows him to "stand" with his feet resting on the base of the unit while he bounces or turns. They have various toys and objects that he can interact with and many also make sounds or play music. They are great for keeping your baby active in a safe environment. These stationary activity centers took the place of walkers that used to be popular, but were extremely dangerous because the baby could move anywhere, potentially even down a flight of stairs. One of the most popular brands of activity centers on the market is the Evenflo ExerSaucers. A few safety considerations to keep in mind are the following:

✳ Read the manufacturer's guidelines on age requirements and follow assembly instructions carefully.

✳ Your baby should be able to hold his head up and have good body control before placing him in an activity center. *Never use pillows or blankets to prop him up!*

✳ Check your activity center often to be sure that none of the toys have become loose or pieces have broken off, and limit the time your baby spends in one.

Bath Tubs

Bathing your baby is always tricky. When they're wet, they are slippery little creatures! A baby bathtub will allow you to bathe her in a safe and clean environment. There are several on the market, but one I love is the Lil' Luxuries Whirlpool, Bubbling Spa & Shower by Summer Infants. This is the ultimate in baby baths. It comes with an infant hammock, allows clean water to constantly circulate through it, and has a temperature gauge and a built-in shower nozzle to make cleaning her off a snap.

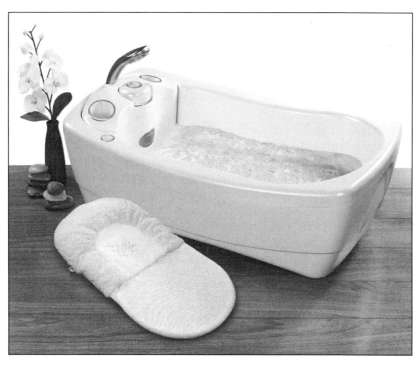

Babies like the spa treatment almost as much as their mothers.

Bathtub rings should never be used in place of a bathtub. Bathtub rings are simply bathing aids used to help babies sit up in the tub and shouldn't be considered a safety device.

While bathtub rings are a great way to make bathing a baby easier, you should never leave your child sitting alone in one. The suction cups on the bottom can become loose, allowing the entire ring to tip forward leaving your baby facedown in the water. Also, a child can slip through the leg holes of the ring and slide down into the water.

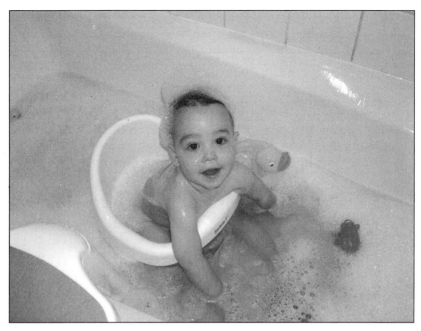

A bathtub ring can provide fun—but *not* safety.

Whenever you bathe your baby, remember these tips:

* **Be organized.** Have everything you need within arm's reach so you never have to take your hand off your baby.

* **Install a tub spout cover.** Babies are extremely slippery when wet—make sure that hard surfaces such as the tub spout are protected. If bathing two children together, be sure that playing does not get out of hand.

* **Keep bath toys clean.** Be sure to allow all bath toys to air dry in a mesh bag and clean them weekly with bleach to prevent mold. An alternative to bleach would be vinegar.

* **Remove adult items from the tub.** Be sure that razors, decorative soaps, candles, glass jars, and other hazardous items are locked away when bathing your baby.

* **Reduce the chance of slips.** Water can get on the floor so be sure you have a rug with a non-skid surface underneath.

* **Never leave your baby unattended for even a moment in the tub!** Keep a cordless phone or cell phone nearby in case of emergencies.

It may seem that, in the blink of an eye, you've gone from looking incredulously at the "positive" line on the pregnancy test to swaddling a baby in your arms and buckling the straps of a high chair or car seat. And yes, there appears to be an inordinate amount of stuff that we Americans feel compelled to buy for our babies. My advice to you is this: keep it as simple as you can, and when shopping for those basic "must-have" products, put safety at the top of your list. While the bells and whistles that come with certain items might increase their aesthetic qualities, they can also present dangers for your little ones. Be vigilant about safety and do your homework to ensure that your baby is as protected as possible.

Chapter 3

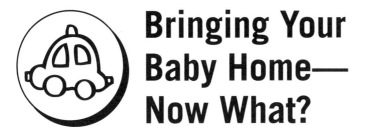

Bringing Your Baby Home— Now What?

I don't know if anyone is completely prepared for the day they first bring their baby home from the hospital. Even "veteran" parents will have some moments of apprehension returning home with their second, third, or fourth baby. The question "What the heck do I know about being a parent?" comes to many parents' minds. After a few days or weeks, however, most parents and children fall into a nice routine, and the rhythm of the family begins. But is your home or the rest of the occupants ready for your baby? Those first few weeks fly by and if you haven't planned ahead of time, you might find yourself dealing with a situation you're not prepared for. Be sure you've got a game plan before you bring your baby home.

There are several truths about parenthood:

* Kids will do things that you never anticipated.

* They will cause you to lose sleep, lose patience, and lose hair.

* You will probably visit an emergency room at least once before your kids turn 18.

* Dinner party conversations that used to revolve around the latest movies and trendy restaurants will now include "war stories" about spit-up, poop, and other baby by-products.

* You will fervently pray for grandkids so that they can torture your kids the way you were tormented.

You Can't Make This Up

Have Tail Will Travel

One day when my daughter was 18 months old, she was happily eating some Cheerios in her high chair, and I decided to go quickly throw in a load of laundry. The laundry room was right off the kitchen so I knew I wouldn't be away from her long. It wasn't more than a few minutes later that I walked back into the kitchen to find she was gone. No, I don't mean she had escaped out of her high chair. She and the high chair were gone! After I recovered from my momentary shock, I heard giggling coming from the den. Our golden retriever must have been walking by her high chair and she had grabbed his tail and held on as he pulled her out of the kitchen into the other room. Since then, I've learned to keep the brakes on my high chair and a bell on my dog!

Sue Carnahan, New York

Do Dogs *Really* Eat Diapers?

I have many friends who would seriously consider their pets more important than their kids. (I'll let them remain anonymous to protect the innocent.) Dogs really are man's best friend, and for many couples, pets were in the picture long before their spouses and certainly their kids. We adopted our first dog Woody about six months before my first son was born. I will admit, that dog was spoiled beyond belief, and he was a great dog—never chewed up anything, listened to commands, and was fairly mellow. I hadn't even considered what Woody's reaction might be when we brought our son home from the hospital the first time. At first, everything seemed fine. He just sniffed the baby's carrier and didn't seem particularly interested. Then I went up to change our son's diaper. All of a sudden, as I'm bending over the changing table, I hear a strange noise and turn around to see Woody raising his leg to pee on the side of the new crib and our brand new carpeting! This from the dog who came completely trained and had **never** before had an accident in our house!

When you decided to start a family, in all likelihood, you didn't run this decision by your dog or cat. And, like me, you might envision one big happy family from the moment you bring your baby home from the hospital. But there's a possibility your pet may feel threatened or stressed. He needs to adjust to big changes in the household and be reassured that he is still loved. It's also hard to admit sometimes, but they are still animals with natural instincts to protect their food and potentially become aggressive if they are teased or threatened in some way.

Unfortunately, we've all heard tragic stories in which a family pet attacked a child. Several years ago, I was hosting a child safety seminar, and one of the attendees was late because she had been at the emergency room with her child. Her son had crawled under a table at the grandfather's house where his 10-year-old Schnauzer was eating. The dog, that had never been aggressive in his life, bit the child on the face.

DID YOU KNOW?   DID YOU KNOW?   DID YOU KNOW?   DID YOU KNOW?

Dog Attacks on Children

When a child less than four years old is the victim of a dog attack, the family dog was the attacker half the time (47%), and the attack almost always happened in the family home. The age group with the second-highest amount of fatalities due to a dog attack are two-year-old children. More than 88 percent of these fatalities occurred when the two-year-old child was left unsupervised with a dog.

Here are some tips to consider in order to make the relationship between your pet and your baby safe and successful right from the beginning:

* **Introduce the pet and baby early.** Make a tape recording of a baby crying and play it occasionally. Bring home a blanket or piece of clothing that the baby has worn so that your dog can get used to her scent immediately.

✴ **Take a few moments to greet your pet when you first come home from the hospital.** Those first few hours when you bring your baby home are exciting and chaotic. The natural inclination might be to put your dog outside or lock him in another room, but this will only make the dog associate the baby with a loss of his special place within the family. Instead, allow your spouse to take the baby for the first few moments so that you can calmly and affectionately greet your dog.

✴ **Never, under any circumstances, leave the dog alone with your baby.** Be sure that anyone taking care of your baby understands this rule and that there is never an exception! Even the most docile and obedient dog could become aggressive or challenge the baby. When you are interacting with your baby and the dog, during diapering, play time, or quiet time, praise the dog and offer him treats so he associates the baby with rewards.

✴ **Create a quiet and safe place for your dog.** You need to find a place that the baby can't access, but also set up some gates to keep your dog out of "off-limit" areas such as the nursery.

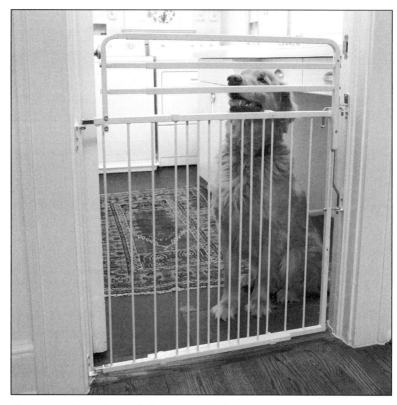

Keep your dog and your baby separated when you are not nearby.

✳ **Establish a protected eating place for your pet.** Make an area where your pet eats that the baby cannot access. In addition to the danger of your child's grabbing the dog's food and being bitten, hard food is a choking hazard for babies and toddlers.

✳ **Don't use stuffed animals as chew toys.** Both your baby and your pet will become confused as to which belongs to whom if they both have stuffed animals as toys. Avoid friendly, but perhaps dangerous, "tug-of-war" games between your dog and your baby.

✳ **Teach your child proper "pet etiquette."** As soon as they're old enough, children should be taught how to treat an animal with respect—no pulling on their tail or other body part, no poking them with a toy or their finger, and always approaching an animal from the front. Kids also need to understand never to corner an animal and to allow them their space. Be sure that the child does not disturb your dog while he's sleeping.

✳ **Install a crib tent.** While it's simply untrue that a cat will suck the air out of a baby's lungs, your pet could snuggle up to your child's face seeking warmth and an infant will not have the ability to turn her head. To be sure that your cat doesn't jump into the crib, you can install a crib tent. Frequently check the mesh on the tent to be sure it's not torn in any way, as once your baby gets older and is standing, it could become a strangulation hazard.

One hazard to keep in mind is "doggie doors." They are a surefire escape method for an inquisitive crawler. A three-year-old can fit through one of these doors and be gone in an instant.

There's Safety in Numbers...Not!

If this isn't your first baby, you'll be facing an entirely different set of issues when bringing your baby home to a big brother or sister. It will be quite easy to become distracted by your infant and overlook potential hazards facing your toddler. There will also be issues of jealously, demands for your attention (oh yeah, from your partner as well!), and the need to divide your time and energy in more ways that you could have ever imagined. They say that a woman loses brain cells every time she has a baby and that they never come back. I believe that, but I also think it's from sheer exhaustion that we misplace items, become complacent about routines, and forget basic facts. This is exactly when accidents occur. Having a second, or third, or fourth baby takes planning and preparation.

While you're pregnant, take some time to teach your older child how to help care for his new baby brother or sister. Establish rules as to when and where he can hold the baby and teach him the proper way to support the baby's head. Explain that he can never pick the baby up out of the crib, car seat, or carrier without your permission. Be sure he understands that he can never try to put anything in the baby's mouth or cover the baby with blankets, pillows, or clothes. Also explain that he should never put anything into the baby's crib such as a blanket, pillow, or stuffed animal.

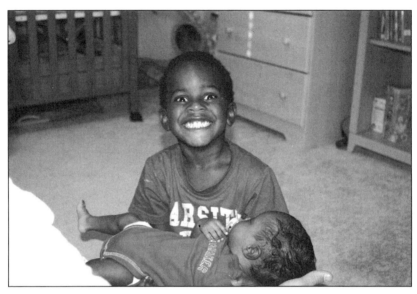

Siblings love to help, so make them a part of your team.

Now that you have more than one, you'll need to review your emergency evacuation plans. Decide who will be in charge of getting each child out of the home in case of a fire or other emergency and establish a meeting location away from the house. It's also a good idea to teach your older child how to dial 911.

It's also time to look at the existing babyproofing items you have in place. As the owner of Safety Mom Solutions babyproofing company, I hear it all the time, "This is our second (or third), and we've already babyproofed." What parents don't usually realize until later is that each baby is different and comes with his or her own unique personality and quirks. I still look at my third and wonder whether they switched her at the hospital—she's so different from her brother and sister.

It's more than likely that your next child will explore different danger zones than those your first discovered. I recall one mother being extremely frustrated as her first would stay exactly where she put her for quite some time, whereas her second baby crawled out the door into the next room before she could even turn around. And, just as new products come on to the market, new safety issues can arise between the time you have your first and second.

✳ **It's important to create a safe zone for your baby.** Unfortunately, an older sibling usually needs access in and out of this area and often will forget to secure a gate. Be sure to install a gate that will self-latch when it swings shut.

✳ **Keep an older sibling's small toys away from the baby.** Store them in covered containers with a photo of them on the outside so that your older child knows what is to be kept in there.

✳ **Visit the Consumer Products Safety Commission Web site (*www.cpsc.gov*) to be sure none of the items that you had for your first baby have been recalled.** Always purchase a new car seat because recent technology has made them safer.

✳ **When getting your children in and out of the car, be sure to teach your older child to keep his hand on the car.** That way, you know he is not running out into a parking lot as you are getting your baby out.

✳ **Place alarms on all windows and doors so that you know if your older child has wandered out while you are tending to your baby.**

Spreading the Love, Not the Germs

Trying to keep your baby healthy with older children around is not easy. Germs are being brought in from school, day care, and other friends' homes. Even before bringing your baby home, begin stressing to your other kids the importance of proper hand washing. Grandparents, friends, and other relatives need to be reminded that proper hand washing is a must, especially for the first few months of a baby's life.

Babies won't begin receiving the vaccines that protect them from a host of viruses until the third month. Common colds that won't necessarily affect adults and older kids can be extremely dangerous to babies and can lead to respiratory syncytial virus (RSV.)

Rate of RSV in the U.S.

Each year, an estimated 125,000 infants in the United States are hospitalized with severe RSV disease, the leading cause of infant hospitalization. Severe RSV infections may cause up to 500 infant deaths annually in the United States.

* RSV can affect any baby, but for those born prematurely or with certain heart or lung conditions, it can be deadly. It's critical that you try to keep your baby as healthy as possible.

* Make sure that everyone washes his or her hands before touching your baby.

* Wipe down "high-touch" surfaces frequently, including light switches, remote controls, refrigerator handles, door knobs, and phones.

* Keep your baby away from anyone who has a cold, fever, or runny nose.

* Don't take your baby to crowded areas, like shopping malls, where there are more people with germs.

* Never allow anyone to smoke around your baby.

* Anyone who will be around your baby should get a flu shot every year.

A Word About SIDS

I'm often asked how I became "The Safety Mom." Unfortunately, my mission was born out of tragedy. In 1997 my first child, Connor, died from Sudden Infant Death Syndrome (SIDS). While I knew about SIDS and had briefly glanced over that section in all the pregnancy books, I never imagined it could happen to me. Fortunately, the rate of SIDS has declined over the past decade, but sadly it's still the leading cause of death for babies one month to one year of age.

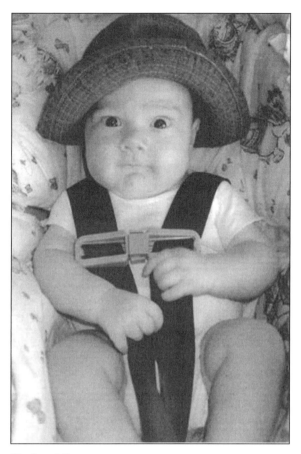

My Angel Connor.

While great strides have been made in determining what causes SIDS, it is still unpredictable and unpreventable. Prior to losing Connor, I was a senior executive at a major public relations firm in Manhattan. My gift was communication. I felt that if I could help spread the word about risk-reduction measures and assist other grieving parents, I would have done something in honor of my son. I took a seat on the Board of Directors for First Candle/SIDS Alliance, and I continue to work to spread the word on risk-reduction measures and offer peer support to other grieving parents. There are a few things to keep in mind:

* SIDS can happen to any baby, regardless of race, sex, and socio-economic factors.

* SIDS is *not* suffocation!

* While risk reductions should be practiced, SIDS is still unpreventable and parents who lose a baby to SIDS need support in overcoming feelings of guilt and responsibility.

Here are some risk-reduction measures that every parent and caregiver must know:

* **Place your baby to sleep on his or her back at nap and nighttime.** This is one of the most important things you can do. Many parents worry that if their baby sleeps on her back, she will aspirate if she spits up. The reality is that she will turn her head to the side. Some parents face pressure from grandparents and older siblings who will insist that their children slept on their tummies, and they were fine. The reality is that, since the Back To Sleep Campaign was implemented in the 1990s, there's been a 50 percent reduction in the rate of SIDS. Still other parents worry about "flat head" and physical development issues. When your baby is awake, provide plenty of "tummy time" for play, but when napping and at night, "back is best!"

* **Don't smoke while you are pregnant and don't let anyone smoke around your baby after he or she is born.** In addition to increasing the risk of SIDS, the harmful effects of secondhand smoke have been clearly documented.

* **Use a safety-approved crib with a firm, tight-fitting mattress covered with only a sheet.** As was discussed in Chapter 2, with the recall of drop-side cribs, parents worry about the safety of cribs, but this is still the safest place for a baby.

* **Remove all soft, fluffy, or loose bedding and toys (including blankets, soft or fluffy bumpers, and positioners).**

* **Use a wearable blanket to replace loose blankets in your baby's crib.**

* **Do not put your baby to sleep on any soft surface (sofas, chairs, waterbeds, quilts, blankets, sheepskins, etc.).**

* **Room sharing is safer than bed sharing.**

* **Do not dress your baby too warm for sleep; keep room temperature between 68 and 72 degrees.**

* **Educate relatives, babysitters and other caregivers about these important safety tips.**

For additional information, visit First Candle/SIDS Alliance's Web site at *www.FirstCandle.org.*

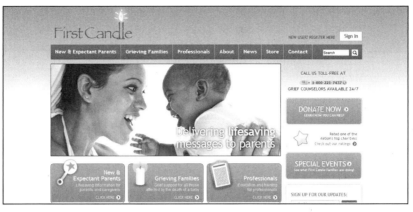

You'll find valuable information at this site.

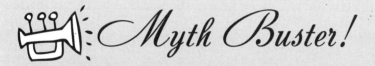

Tummy vs. Back Sleeping

Myth: It's dangerous to have babies sleep on their backs because they could die if they spit up or vomit while they're asleep.

For healthy, full-term babies there is no greater risk for choking while lying on their backs than there is when lying on their stomachs. The United States Department of Health and Human Services states: "Healthy babies automatically swallow or cough up fluids. There has been no increase in choking or other problems for babies who sleep on their backs." The American Academy of Pediatrics also states that there is no evidence that choking is more frequent among infants lying on their backs.

Postpartum Depression

While some people discount it, postpartum depression is a clinical diagnosis and can be debilitating and dangerous. From mothers who have murdered their children, such as Andrea Yates, to celebrities like Brooke Shields, it is the high-profile cases of postpartum depression that make the news. Yet every year approximately 15 percent of new moms suffer from postpartum depression. Partners and grandparents might try to discount postpartum depression as a case of the "baby-blues," but it's different. Baby blues, which can include feelings of sadness, being overwhelmed, loss of appetite, and difficulty sleeping, go away after a few weeks. Postpartum depression, however, lasts longer, and the symptoms are more severe. Women who suffer from postpartum depression can have thoughts of hurting themselves or their baby, don't feel that they can care for their baby, and can barely function throughout the day. Unfortunately, some women never talk about these feelings because they are afraid no one will understand, or they think it makes them a bad mother. They feel embarrassed, ashamed, or guilty about feeling depressed when they are supposed to be happy.

It's impossible to predict who will have postpartum depression, but researchers believe it can be caused by a dramatic change in hormone levels. Women who have a history of depression are also more susceptible.

The important thing to recognize is that if you have feelings of sadness, depression, you find yourself constantly crying or unable to eat, or you feel you can't take care of your baby, talk to your doctor immediately. Go online to find chat rooms and blogs discussing postpartum depression so that you realize you're not the only one having these feelings and ask your partner and family for help.

What's Your Escape Plan?

How many of us have *really* thought about an escape plan in the event of a fire or other emergency in our home? Even if you and your partner have the best relationship in the world, you might be inclined to think "every man for himself" if something were to happen. But once a baby comes along, everything changes. Then you'd lay down your life to save that precious being. But there's a reason the airlines instruct parents to put on their oxygen masks before their child's. If you're rendered unconscious, you'll be no help to anyone. So, sit down and have "the talk." In the event of a fire, tornado, earthquake, or some other natural disaster, who would get the baby? Do you have a meeting place outside the home? What if you and your spouse were both at work and the baby was at day care or with a babysitter? How many of us have actually read the instructions on our fire extinguisher? Would you know how to use yours in a fire? Not only do you have to consider these things, but you also need to rehearse the various scenarios. Just as they have fire drills in schools, it's important to practice your home emergency plan and have emergency supplies on hand.

I lived through the Northridge earthquake in Southern California in 1994, long before I had kids. I was young, and didn't have a clue about owning an emergency preparedness kit. After that, my roommate and I put together a box of emergency supplies, gallons of water, some non-perishable food, batteries, and so on. When I moved back to New York, I didn't bother putting together a new kit—it just sort of fell by the wayside. Then 9/11 happened. I was working in New York City at the time, but fortunately that day was my one day per week to work at home in the suburbs. My son was three at the time, and he was at day care a few miles from our house. After the first plane hit the towers and the news reports started coming in, I knew, being that close to Manhattan, that panic and chaos would start in the surrounding areas. I knew we had to get my son, get some cash, and get some supplies before food ran out in the stores. At that point, no one knew what to expect. I don't think anyone could have anticipated or planned for that day, but it gave everyone, especially people who lived in the affected areas, a different perspective on emergency preparedness. Now, not only do we have emergency plans for our home, but also we know what we would do if we were away from our house and the kids were at school. We have emergency kits in our home and in our car. Being prepared also means taking the appropriate safety precautions and having systems in place to keep our home as safe as possible.

Here are some additional tips to keep in mind:

* **Having properly installed smoke alarms cuts the chances of dying in a reported fire by half.** Install smoke alarms in every bedroom, outside every sleeping area, and on every level of the home. Ideally, these alarms should be wired so that if one goes off, it will cause the others to sound as well. Consider purchasing one with a built-in escape light. Make a note on the calendar to test the smoke alarm on the first day of every month.

* **Be sure to place specially designed stickers from the fire department on the window of each child's bedroom.** This safety feature will alert firefighters that a child could be present in that room.

* **Keep fire extinguishers in various places around your home, including the kitchen, garage, near the furnace, and near any fireplace.**

* **If you are using a portable space heater, be sure it has built-in safety features, such as automatic shutoffs, anti-tipping devices, and heat guards.**

* **When you have small children in the home, install a baby gate around the fireplace to prevent access.**

* **Purchase a 2-Story Emergency Fire Escape Ladder and keep it somewhere in or near your bedroom.**

* **Teach your children never to try and put out a fire themselves, but to leave the house immediately and call 911 from a neighbor's home.** Have a fire drill once every few months so that everyone can practice.

✻ **Create a first aid kit to keep in your home and your car.** This kit should include Band-Aids, a thermometer, ice pack/heat pack, children's and adult acetaminophen, children's and adult ibuprofen, tweezers, antihistamine such as Benadryl, a first-aid/antibiotic ointment such as Neosporin, antiseptic wipes, a breathing barrier for performing CPR, and a pair of latex gloves.

✻ **Along with a first aid kit, you should have a disaster preparedness kit.** This can be a large, sturdy plastic box with a tight lid and should include jugs of water, batteries, flashlights, blankets, canned food, a can opener, a Swiss Army knife, and bandages.

Carbon Monoxide: The Silent Killer

In addition to smoke alarms, carbon monoxide (CO) alarms also need to be installed. As an odorless, invisible, tasteless gas, carbon monoxide can be particularly harmful. In fact, according to the Centers for Disease Control for 1999–2004, "Unintentional CO exposure accounts for an estimated 15,000 emergency department visits and 500 unintentional deaths in the United States each year."

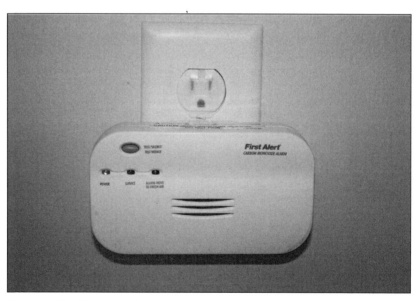

Products like First Alert Carbon Monoxide Detector *will* save lives.

Carbon monoxide gases can build up from furnaces, wood-burning stoves, attached garages, and other areas with heating units in the home. Unfortunately, only about one-third of homes in the country have CO detectors installed. Be sure to mount the detectors on every level of the house and outside every sleeping area. Because a fair number of deaths from carbon monoxide poisoning occur with those who are asleep, the Journal for the American Medical Association (JAMA) recommends CO detectors that emit an alarm loud enough to wake someone. In 2010, five college students died in a Florida motel room from CO poisoning when they inadvertently left their car running in the garage under their room.

Many people ignore their CO alarms when they sound, assuming that it's a false alarm. This could be a deadly mistake. CO poisoning can come on without you realizing it. Symptoms include nausea, shortness of breath, headaches, confusion, dizziness, or fainting. If anyone is experiencing any of these symptoms you should immediately call 911 and leave the house instantly. The local fire department will be called to come in and assess the source of the CO. There was an incident several years ago in which an elderly woman's CO detector sounded. Her system was tied into ADT Home Security Systems so a responder called her home to check and informed the woman that firefighters had already been dispatched to her home. The woman insisted that nothing was wrong and was adamant that it was a false alarm. She refused to let the firefighters into her home when they arrived. The diligent responder kept the woman on the phone until she was convinced to let the firefighters in to check. The fire department team quickly determined that the levels were so high that the woman had approximately two hours left before she was unconscious and probably would have died from the toxic gases.

Keep in mind that the detectors are intended to gauge levels that would be harmful to a healthy adult. Babies, kids, older adults, and anyone with respiratory problems may be more susceptible to even low levels of carbon monoxide. Most CO alarms have an average shelf life of two years, so be sure to test yours regularly to make sure it is working properly.

Your CO detector should have a battery backup in case you lose power. The easiest solution is to get combination smoke detectors/CO detectors so you don't have to worry about two separate devices.

Preparing your home, your pet, and any siblings for the arrival of a baby takes some planning and a small amount of effort to ensure that the transition is safe and a little less chaotic. Most new parents aren't prepared for the sheer exhaustion of caring for an infant and the sleep deprivation that is inevitably a part of the first few weeks and months. It's easy for accidents to happen when you're in this state, so be as ready as possible for all scenarios.

Chapter 4

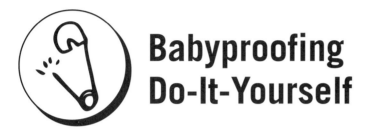

Babyproofing Do-It-Yourself

Babyproofing is one of those items that goes on the "Honey-Do" list and gets ignored for quite some time. Whether it's a matter of not being the handiest person on the block or just being in a sense of denial over really needing to do it, most people (especially men) figure that the baby won't be crawling for a long time, so they can put off babyproofing for another day. The reality is that your baby will start crawling when you least expect it, so be prepared. No place is too small or too large to put some safeguards into place.

You've probably read or heard that you should get down on your hands and knees and crawl around to see what hazards might lurk around your home. I personally find this advice ridiculous. It assumes that a baby thinks like a logical and rational adult. Last time I looked around, I didn't notice a grown man sticking paper clips in electrical outlets or pulling the flat screen TV down on his head (although I'm sure he might consider it after a disappointing loss by his favorite NFL team).

For many first-time parents, there are hazards they would never see or consider. As the saying goes, kids do the darndest things! It's a worthwhile investment to hire a professional babyproofer to come in and assess what needs to be done. To find a reputable professional in your area, visit the International Association for Child Safety Web site at *www.iafcs.com*. Babyproofers who are members are required to meet certain criteria and go through a certification process that qualifies them to perform consultations and install products. Most babyproofers will offer a consultation and then provide you with a list of items that should be installed. You can then choose whether to do each project yourself or hire the company to do some of the jobs. My company, Safety Mom Solutions (*www.safetymomsolutions.com*), serves the New York, Connecticut, and northern New Jersey areas

You Can't Make This Up

A Creative Use for Crayons

My son was about 18 months old and was being very quiet—the kind of quiet where you know he has to be up to something. That quiet. I went into the room, and he was standing in front of the TV. I walked away, and my "Mommy Sense" kicked in. I returned to find him shoving crayons into the small hole that was left when our power button broke. (It was about the size of a dime.) My husband took apart the TV and found 62 crayons in the bottom! I'm so happy I found him in the act or the TV would have melted the crayons and either broken the TV or caught on fire.

Dana S., Pittsburgh, PA

Gates

The most important item to have in place are gates. For someone who is handy, this might be something you can tackle yourself, but keep in mind that gates are often tricky. Unless you are installing a gate onto two flat surfaces, it may be difficult. There are several types of gates:

✻ Hardware-mounted

✻ Pressure-mounted

✻ Pressure-mounted walk-through

✻ Sectional

✻ Fireplace gates

✻ Retractable

Hardware-Mounted Gates

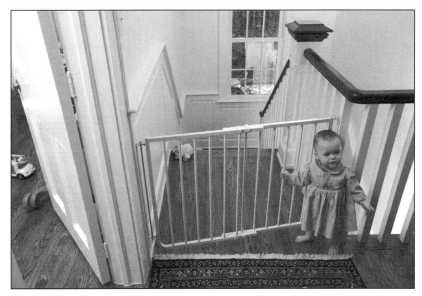

Cardinal Stairway Special Safety gate.
Photo courtesy of Cardinal Gates

Hardware-mounted gates are the best and most commonly used. They are the *only* gates that should be used at the top of the stairs. A gate at the top of a staircase is the most critical one that you will install and *must* be hardware mounted. It needs to be drilled and attached to both sides of the gate location. Here are a few things to look for:

* A gate that's easy to use with one-handed operation.

* A safety mechanism that prevents it from opening out over the stairs and will only allow it to open toward you.

* Some of these gates are self-latching, which means you will not have to turn around to close the gate. Simply swing the gate behind you until it hits the latch, and it will lock itself.

Pressure-Mounted Walk-Through Gates

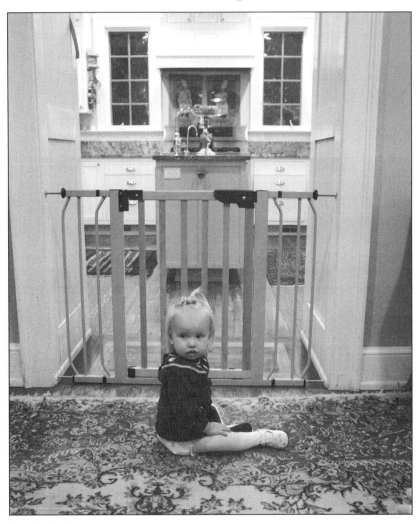

Cardinal AutoLock pressure gate.
Photo courtesy of Cardinal Gates

The pressure-mounted walk-through gate is an extremely popular style of gate because it can be installed in a few minutes without the use of special tools. As its name implies, it adjusts to the width of the opening to tighten against two solid wall surfaces. These gates should *never* be used at the top of the stairs. They are generally used in low traffic areas that aren't often entered.

While they are easy to install and relatively convenient to use, these gates do have drawbacks. Each time you walk through the gate, you will need to turn around and realign it to lock it. If you have a baby or packages in your arms, this may not be easy to do.

All pressure-mounted gates will loosen over time, depending upon how frequently they are used, so they need to be checked often and adjusted as necessary. Also, the bar under the portion of the gate that opens to maintain the pressure can be a tripping hazard.

Pressure-Mounted Gates

Pressure-mounted gates are similar in all respects to pressure-mounted walk-through gates, but are one solid piece. This gate is extremely inconvenient since it must be removed and replaced or stepped over to access the other side. With a baby in your arms, not only is it unsafe, but it's virtually impossible to remove and replace. And it won't take a toddler long to figure out he can use a chair or bench to climb over it just like mommy and daddy do! This is, however, the perfect gate to use at grandma's house or another frequently visited place, where there is a room that is completely off-limits.

Sectional Gates for Wide or Irregular Openings

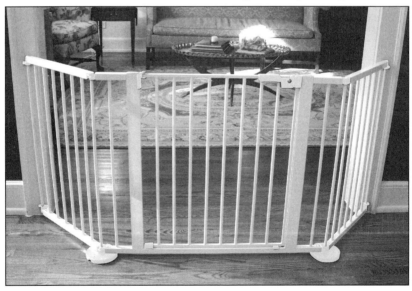

Cardinal VersaGate.
Photo courtesy of Cardinal Gates

These gates are extremely versatile because they can be used to cover wide openings, make turns, or be attached together to form a play area. They are strongest when used at an angle or with a bend, and with additional extensions, can expand to be as long as you need.

Hearth Gates

Hearth gates are specifically designed to go around fireplaces and wood-burning stoves, but can also be used around barbeques. They're intended to protect your child from the fire, as well as the hard edges around the hearth. Similar to a sectional gate, it can be bent and adjusted to go around a fireplace.

Retractable Gates

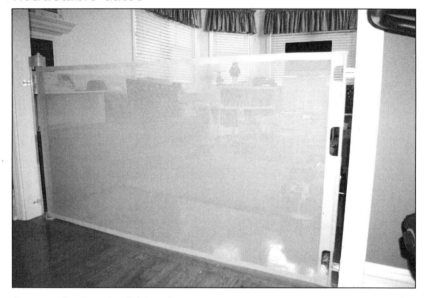

An example of a retractable gate.

These gates are retractable and can be rolled up into a cylinder so they are out of the way when not in use.

Wood Versus Metal Gates

Most gates are metal or plastic, but there are some wood gates on the market available in various finishes to match your stair rail. Keep in mind that wood gates are harder to keep clean and can swell or shrink slightly with heat and humidity. Wood gates also need more frequent adjustments than metal gates.

Installation How-To's

Important: All gates need to have flat wood planes (such as a doorway) to be installed properly. If those don't exist, they will need to be created to install a gate.

Materials That Might Be Required for Installation

✻ Wood rails made of maple or poplar 3/4" thick by 1 1/2" wide. Thicker rails can be used, if necessary.

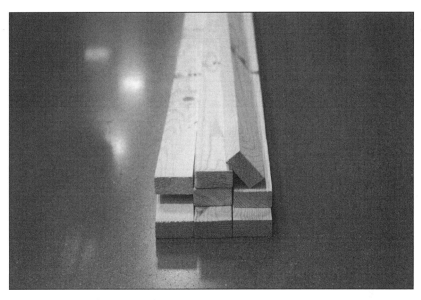

Wood rails used for installation.

✻ Gate extensions.

✻ Baluster mounting kit: Gives you the ability to mount a child safety gate between two wood or metal balusters (the spindles at a staircase). It's an ideal solution if you are installing a baby gate when you can't attach your safety gate to a newel post.

✻ No hole mounting kit: Allows gate installation to a newel post (vertical banister post) without drilling into it.

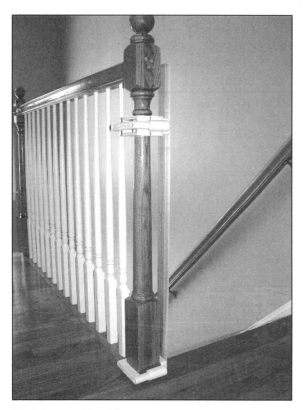

No hole mounting kit.
Photo courtesy of KidCo, Inc.

Hardware-Mounted Gates

It is a good idea to assemble the gate and place it in the intended location. This can help you decide the side on which to hinge it and determine any problems that may arise. Verify the attachment points and choose which side of the railing on which to attach the gate. Keep in mind where the gate will be if it is left open. In general, gates are attached to the side of the doorway closest to the wall. This way they won't stick into the middle of a room. Instructions for installation are as follows:

1. Assemble gate following instructions provided. Use gate template if provided.
2. Measure and mark holes.
3. Attach hinge and gate.
4. Attach latch.
5. Adjust gate so it latches properly.
6. Place 1" Velcro square on gate anywhere it hits walls/doorways.

7. Adjust gate so that it is level.

8. Mark locking mechanism on opposite side.

9. Pre-drill holes for latch.

Stairway Installs

Gates installed at the top of the stairs should have a special safety bracket or mechanism that prevents them from opening out over the stairs. Most often, stairway gates are attached with the hinged side to the wall and the latch side to the post. Instructions for installation are as follows:

1. Assemble the gate.

2. Hold at the top step. You do not want the gate to be out over the step in any way. You also want the gate to be straight across the step.

3. Mark the hinged side and measure up 7" to mark the first hole.

4. Check for studs.

5. Install the wood rail, if necessary, and attach the hinge to the rail/wall/doorway.

6. Attach the gate to the hinge.

7. Use a level to make sure the gate is level.

8. Extend the gate to the proper size.

9. Mark the gate contact point on the latch side.

10. Install the post kit/baluster kit/wood rail, if necessary.

11. Mark the latch holes and pre-drill.

12. Attach the latch.

13. Adjust the gate so it latches well and is secure.

14. You can use Velcro squares on the latch to cut down metal-on-metal noise and on the gate itself where it hits the wall.

15. Lean hard on the gate to be sure it's secure and can withstand a child pushing on it.

Gates at the bottom of the stairs will follow the same instructions as those for the top of the stairs. Sometimes, the gate at the bottom of the stairs will need to be installed one or two steps up to achieve a cleaner, more secure install. Many staircases have radius banisters that make a bottom step install more difficult.

Special Situations (Balusters and Rails)

If your balusters don't seem sturdy you can install a rail:

1. Measure from the top of the step to the railing.

2. Cut the wood rail.

3. Toe screw (screw at an angle through rail and into floor) or use a small L-bracket to secure the rail to the floor.

4. Use an L-bracket to secure the wood rail to the underside of the railing.

If you have a wrought iron or metal staircase, there are several options. A baluster kit can be installed or a wood rail can be attached in two different ways:

1. Cut the wood rail to the proper size and sand the edges.

2. Use heavy-duty adhesive tape between the rail and the metal/iron post.

3. Drill through the wood rail from side to side in several locations.

4. Use zip ties through the rail and then around the metal/iron post and tighten.

5. The zip ties and adhesive tape will hold the wood rail in place.

Or, if you are willing to drill into the metal post, follow these instructions:

1. Cut the wood rail to the proper size.

2. You can use heavy-duty adhesive tape between the rail and the metal/iron post to hold the rail in place.

3. Drill several holes with the metal drill bit.

4. Using the proper size tek screws, attach the wood rail to the post.

Installing a hardware-mounted gate can become frustrating if certain problems arise. Here are solutions for the most common problems.

No Studs in Wall or Difficult-to-Find Studs

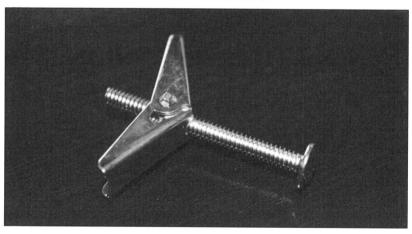

A toggle bolt.

Use these directions to put in a toggle bolt.

1. Use a toggle bolt to secure the rail.
2. Drill holes for toggle bolts in the rail.
3. Hold the rail in place and mark the holes on the wall.
4. Drill proper sized holes in the wall.
5. Place the toggle bolt in the rail.
6. Attach the toggle.
7. Secure it to the wall.
8. Plaster and lathe the walls.

Brick or Cement Walls

Use tapcons or concrete anchors with masonry bits to secure the rail.

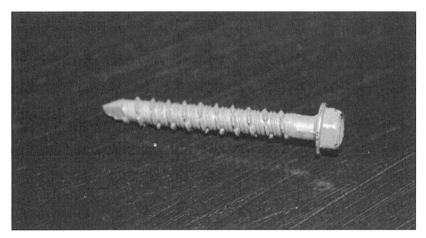

A tapcon.

Baseboard in the Way

Use a wood rail attached to the wall to bring everything out to the same plane.

If the baseboard is too high or there is molding/wainscoting in the way, follow these steps:

1. Use a thicker rail (about 1 1/2" thick).
2. Hold the rail in place.
3. Mark obstructions on the rail with a pencil.
4. Use a jigsaw or sander to notch the rail.
5. Attach the rail to the wall.

Installing a Newel Post Kit

1. Insert the wood blocks into the clamps.
2. Place the clamp on the bottom of the newel post close to the floor.
3. Tighten with the screws provided, but do not overtighten.
4. Place the top clamp on the post.
5. The height of the top clamp will depend on the gate you are using. Most gates are approximately 30" and need 2" of ground clearance.
6. Insert the round post adapters, if necessary.
7. Attach the wood rail to the clamps. The height of the wood rail also depends on the gate you are using.
8. Use a level to plumb the wood rail.
9. Place a level on the face of the rail. Use shims provided, if necessary, to plumb the rail.
10. Attach the gate.

How to Deal with a Spiral Staircase

In most cases, a gate between the posts at the bottom of a spiral staircase will still leave access to the stairs from behind or the side. The entire stairway needs to be closed off. The best solution is a sectional gate.

1. Choose two attachment points that close off all access to the stairs.
2. Attach the gate and the appropriate extensions.

You can follow the installation directions for a regular hardware-mounted gate install for the top of the stairs, as long as the railings and balusters have the proper spacing and protection. If the railings present a problem, you can follow the same install pattern for the bottom of a spiral staircase and block off all access.

Sectional Gates

This gate is used for wide doorway openings.

1. Assemble the gate following instructions to a measurement as close to the door opening as possible.
2. If the gate is larger than the opening, you can angle the gate at the sectional breaks to make the gate smaller. Putting a slight bend in the gate actually makes the gate stronger. For example, KidCo configure gates are 6' long. They have extensions at 8" and 24". Every 2', there is a sectional break. This is the point at which you can put a slight bend in the gate. If the opening is 7' and you are using a gate and two 8" extensions, the gate will be slightly larger

than the opening. Bend the gate a little at the sections on either side of the section that opens until the gate fits the opening.

3. Attach the gate to the doorframe.

Windows

Falls are the leading cause of unintentional injury in the home. According to the National SAFE KIDS Campaign, approximately 18 children ages 10 and under die annually from falls from windows. Another 4,700 children ages 14 and under will require treatment each year for window fall–related injuries.

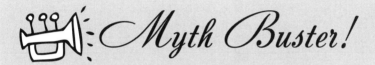

Deaths Due to Short Falls

Myth: Short falls can't kill a baby.

There has been significant controversy over the years as to whether short falls could actually cause enough trauma to a baby's brain to cause death. Many pediatricians over the past several decades have testified in cases of potential "Shaken Baby Syndrome" that a short fall could not possibly cause the damage seen in these babies. Yet in 2001, Dr. John Plunkett, a physician from Minnesota, disproved this theory in an article that included the videotaped fall of a toddler from a 28-inch high indoor play set that resulted in the toddler's death two days later. There is now a growing body of evidence that, indeed, even short falls can cause death.

Regardless of whether they are on the first floor or fifth, all windows should be safeguarded. People may mistakenly believe that screens are sufficient protection, but screens will not prevent a child from falling through a window! Furniture and items on which kids can stand should be removed from underneath windows.

There are various types of windows, including single hung, double hung, sliding, and casement. Each requires different products to secure them. Double hung are the most common and open vertically from the top and bottom. If the window opens only from the bottom and the top is stationary, it is single hung. Whenever possible, double-hung windows should be opened from the top, not the bottom. If they must be opened from the bottom, open them no more than four inches.

These windows can be secured with the Window Wedge by Cresci Products (wedge locks work only with wood windows). Or you can use window stops or a BurglaBar (*www.addalock.com*), which is an adhesive mount flip lock.

Both Guardian Angel and KidCo make guards that will work for casement windows. Even if you do have guards, windows should still be kept locked at all times.

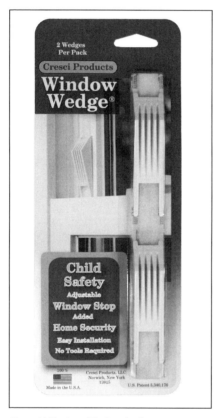

Cresci Window Wedge locks.

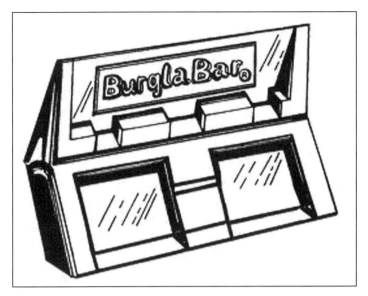

BurglaBar *www.addalock.com*

Without a doubt, window guards are the best and safest option for securing your window. In New York City, window guards are required for any building that has three or more apartments and where a child under 10 years of age lives. Every window must have a guard except for those leading to a fire escape. Window guards screw into the frames of the windows and have bars spaced four inches apart. They stay affixed to the window at all times, but can be easily removed in the event of an emergency. There are several manufacturers including Guardian Angel (*www.angelguards.com*) and Looking Glass Window Guard (*www.lookingglasswindowguard.com*).Window guards should be used in conjunction with window stops or window wedges for the greatest protection.

Installation How-To's

Window Wedges

1. Place Velcro on both sides of top section of window.

2. Open window no more than four inches.

3. Attach the wedge to Velcro at the top of window.

BurglaBars

This is for use on double hung, sliding, and shower or glass doors.

1. Determine the location.
2. Leave enough room to flip the lock into an open position.
3. Clean the surface with rubbing alcohol.
4. Attach the lock.
5. Leave open for 24 hours for the adhesive to cure.

Wedge Locks and Window Stops

1. Determine the location.
2. Hold the lock or stop in place and mark with a pencil.
3. Pre-drill the holes for the screw.
4. Attach with the screws provided.

Sliding Window Locks

Here's how to attach a sliding window lock.

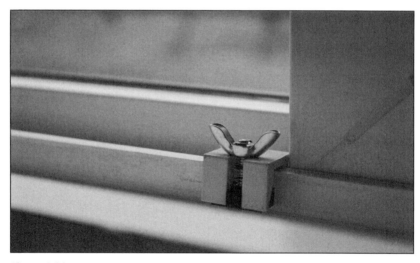

Figure 4.11
Sliding window lock.

1. Attach the lock to the track.
2. Drop the groove in the lock over the track the window slides in. The wing nut is the screw that holds the lock in place. The lock should be placed right behind the window or in a location so that the window can open no more than four inches.
3. Tighten down the lock with the wing nut provided.

Window Guards

1. Measure the horizontal distance inside the window frame to determine the appropriate window guard. It's important that you use the correct size window guard.

2. For casement windows, measure both horizontally and vertically. Consult with the manufacturer to determine whether the guard can be installed vertically to protect the window or if you need to purchase two guards to stack horizontally in order to cover the entire window.

3. Guards can be mounted inside or on the front of the window frame.

4. Be certain that the wood you are drilling into is not rotted.

5. Place the guard on the window.

6. Mark the holes and pre-drill.

7. Secure the window guard using the screws provided.

8. Once installed, check that the guards are completely secure and do not move in any direction.

Window Blind Cords

Window coverings with cords pose a serious risk for children. In the past few years, over five million Roman Shades, roller and roll-up blinds, and vertical and horizontal blinds have been recalled due to strangulation hazards.

DID YOU KNOW? DID YOU KNOW? DID YOU KNOW? DID YOU KNOW?

Cord Blind Injuries

According to the Window Covering Safety Council, approximately 200 infants and children have died due to cords from window coverings since 1990. Window blinds, corded shades, and draperies manufactured before 2001 should be replaced immediately.

The risk with Roman Shades or similar window coverings is that children can place an exposed inner cord around their neck and then have it become entangled with the loops. Whether it's in your home or that of your child's caregiver or another relative, if there are shades with cords, it's important to tie them up and out of the way. This can be done by installing window cord cleats and window cord stops. Also, be sure that cribs and other furniture are positioned away from any window cords.

Installation How-To's

Cord Cleats

1. Choose the cord side of the window.
2. Determine the height of the top cleat.
3. Mark the holes.
4. Pre-drill.
5. Attach with the screws provided.
6. Place second cleat 6" to 10" below top cleat.
7. Attach second cleat.

Looped Blind Cords

Install a proper tie-down device so that the cord is taught but still functions. A tie-down device can be several things. Most blind stores will actually sell them if they are not already provided with the blinds. Often, the tie-down device is on the looped cord, just not secured. Any kind of clamp can be used.

Drawers/Cabinets Locks

Kids love to explore and one of their favorite games is pulling everything they can out of cabinets and drawers. I'm so disorganized that often my kids will discover something I misplaced months earlier so this is sometimes a benefit. But there are many cabinets and drawers that hold dangerous items that need to be kept locked away. There are several ways to secure cabinets, depending on the style and material. There are also pros and cons to each lock:

* Adhesive mount cabinet locks are easy to install but not as durable as other locks. If this is your last or only child and you'll need them for only a few months or a year, this may work.

* Exterior cabinet locks, such as sliding cabinet locks are difficult to operate and accessible to kids.

* Magnetic cabinet locks such as Tot-Locks or KidCo Adhesive/ Hardware-mount magnetic locks are harder to install.

* One-piece or swivel locks are easy to install and very durable.

* One-piece spring latches are easy to install and fairly durable.

* Wonder Latch brand is easy to install and mounts where others won't.

These locks can be installed in built-in kitchen cabinets, bathroom vanities, and most pieces of furniture.

In order to install locks effectively, you must first determine what sort of drawer you have:

    ✱ Overlay drawers are the most common. These are ones in which the door and drawer faceplates lie over the cabinet frame. They are the easiest in which to install a lock.

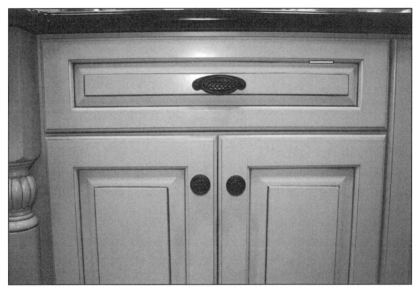

Example of overlay cabinets.

    ✱ Flush drawers are ones in which the door and drawer faceplates recess into the cabinet frame.

Installation How-To's

Interior Hardware-Mounted Cabinet Lock

Here's a good way to keep kids out of a cabinet.

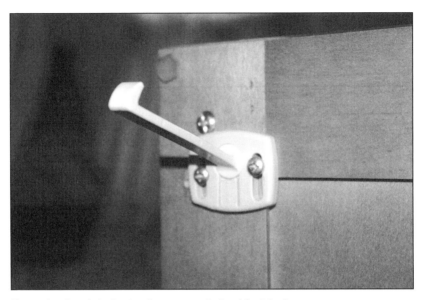

Example of an interior hardware-mounted cabinet lock.
Image provided by KidSafeInc.com

1. Center the lock on the drawer.
2. Mark the holes on the lock and latch and drill with a drill bit slightly smaller than the screw provided. This will ensure that the wood of the cabinet frame will not split or crack.
3. Attach the lock with the screws provided.
4. Close the drawer and mark the lock on the cabinet frame.
5. Remove the drawer.
6. Attach the catch where the lock hits the cabinet frame.
7. Re-install the drawer.
8. Adjust lock on drawer, if necessary.

Lock on a Flush Frame Drawer

If a drawer is recessed and on the same plane as the framing, nothing can be mounted to the frame. Therefore, the catch cannot be mounted as normal because the drawer will not close all the way.

Follow the previous steps to attach the lock and then follow the instructions below:

1. When attaching the catch, mount a small block of wood to the backside of the cabinet frame where the lock hits. The block should be installed where the lock that is mounted on the drawer will pass under the frame. The block generally needs to be ³/₄"

thick and about 1" wide (size may differ depending on the size of the cabinet frame between the drawers) and 3" long.

2. Remove the drawer.

3. Use a spring clamp to hold the block in place on the frame.

4. Reach inside the cabinet and drill through the block to be mounted and slightly into the cabinet frame. Be careful not to drill all the way through the face of the frame.

5. Attach the block with the appropriate size screws.

6. Keep the block flush with the bottom of the frame.

7. Attach the catch to the block.

8. Reinstall the drawer.

9. Adjust the lock if necessary.

Lock on a Door

1. Place the lock on the side of the door that opens.

2. Make sure the lock placement will still allow the door to close.

3. The lock should be slightly below the cabinet frame to allow room for the catch.

4. Mark the lock.

5. Pre-drill the holes.

6. Attach the lock.

7. Mark the lock on the frame.

8. Attach the catch.

9. Adjust the lock if necessary.

Lock on a Flush Frame Door

1. Follow the previous steps to attach the lock.

2. When attaching the catch, mount a small block of wood to the backside of the cabinet frame where the lock hits.

3. Keep the block flush with the bottom of the frame.

4. Attach the catch to the block.

5. Adjust the lock if necessary.

One-Piece Lock in Drawer

1. Center the lock in the drawer.

2. Make sure the lock will catch the cabinet framing.

3. Mark the holes and pre-drill.

4. Attach the lock.

5. Adjust the lock, if necessary.

One-Piece Lock on Door

1. Place the lock on the side of the door that opens.
2. Make sure the lock placement will still allow the door to close.
3. Make sure the lock will catch the cabinet framing.
4. Mark the holes and pre-drill.
5. Attach the lock.
6. Adjust the lock, if necessary.
7. If there is no room for a cabinet lock on the inside of a drawer, a Wonder latch can be mounted on the outside of the drawer.

Wonder Latch Install

The Wonder Latch can work wonders.

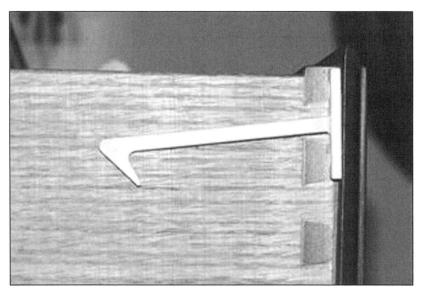

The Wonder Latch.
Photo courtesy of BabyPro.com

1. Hold the latch in position, making sure the drawer will still close.
2. Mark the holes.
3. Pre-drill.
4. Attach with the screws provided.
5. Mark the latch location on the frame and pre-drill.
6. Partially sink the screw into the side of the frame.
7. The latch will catch the screw to prevent the drawer from opening.

In certain instances, the cabinet and drawers will need to be retrofitted to accommodate the locks. Below are some scenarios in which this might be the case:

If there is no framing for the catch, you need to install a wood rail.

1. Measure the interior of the cabinet.
2. Cut the wood rail to size.
3. Install the wood rail where the catch needs to be.

If the drawer/door face is too thick and the lock is not long enough, follow this information:

❋ Stack extra bases or blocks behind the lock where it attaches to the drawer/door to extend the cabinet lock.

Doors

I'll never forget when my son was just four years old, I was downstairs doing laundry, and he was upstairs playing. In no more time than it takes to fold a load of clothes, I came back upstairs to find that he wasn't in the playroom where I had left him. I started calling for him and there was no answer. It didn't take long for me to panic as I ran frantically through the house looking for him. No doors were open, but I decided to go outside to check if he had wandered out to the swing set. When I didn't see him there, I started screaming his name. All of a sudden, I heard him very cheerily call out, "Here I am, Mom!" My little four-year-old had wandered next door to visit the neighbors who were grilling outside on their deck. I'm sure my neighbors thought I was the shrew of the century as I marched over there, grabbed his arm, and summarily dragged him home.

Toddlers are escape artists and will demonstrate their abilities quite often. A few summers ago, my friend rented a vacation home on the Jersey shore. One day, her husband was out entertaining their two older children while she stayed home napping with her toddler. She awoke a half hour later to find a police officer standing in her rental home with her son. As she was napping, he had woken up, wandered outside, and was sitting on the sidewalk in front of the house. Fortunately, someone driving by saw him and alerted the police. But imagine her horror when she awoke!

All doors to the outside of the house should have an additional lock (safety chain, deadbolt) up high enough so that a child cannot reach them. Automatic door closers are great additional layers of safety for keeping certain doors closed. They can be used on doors leading to garages, attics, or basement doors in order to protect access to the stairs, especially when there are older children in the house and the basement is a playroom.

There are rooms inside the home that should be off-limits to toddlers; the doors to these rooms also require additional locks. Exercise rooms, media rooms, and home offices are all examples of high-supervision areas that are especially dangerous for kids. Any lockable door knob in the interior of the house should have the proper emergency door key nearby (the top of the door jamb is the best place) in case a toddler locks himself in from the inside. There are various locks that can be used on these doors, and they include surface bolts, flip locks, chain door guards, top-of-door locks, bi-fold locks, and shutter bars.

Installation How-To's

Automatic Door Closers—Solid and Metal Doors

If you're unsure whether your door is hollow, tap on it and pay attention to how it sounds and feels. Hollow-core doors are usually slab doors, meaning they are completely flat and very light. An install template is included with the closers.

1. Determine the side on which the closer goes. The closer will go on the hinged side of the door.
2. Determine the door type and choose the appropriate hardware, either wood or metal.
3. Cut out the template, mark the holes using the template, and pre-drill.
4. Assemble the door closer.
5. Attach the door closer to the door and close the door.
6. Attach the arm to the jamb.
7. Adjust the speed of the closer to your liking.

Automatic Door Closers—Hollow Doors

If you have a hollow-core door, the automatic door closer should be thru-bolted. Hollow-core doors have only a small wood framing around the edge of the door, and the door itself is only $1/4$" thick. In this case, the screws will pull during the install process. Thru-bolting means drilling all the way through the door and then using a bolt with nuts and washers to hold the door closer onto the door.

1. Using the template provided, drill completely through the door.
2. Replace the hardware with bolts, nuts, and washer.
3. Attach the door closer to the door. This will secure the closer.
4. On hollow-core doors, you can also use a surface mount spring door closer. These small, one-piece cylinders attach to the door casing (the molding around the door) and have a small arm to spring the door back to the closed position. These are cheaper and easier to install, but will only work on light doors.

Front-Mount Door Closer

1. Determine the location on the hinged side of the door.
2. Mark holes and pre-drill.
3. Attach the door closer.
4. Adjust the arm, using the Allen wrench provided to desired speed.

Surface Bolts

These can be used to lock all doors, and they come in a variety of finishes to match your hardware. They can be placed either vertically or horizontally on your door and should be placed within reach of adults, but out of reach of children.

1. Mark the holes where the surface bolt will be mounted and pre-drill the holes.
2. Attach the bolt using the screw provided.
3. The locking plate is attached to the door jamb opposite the bolt.
4. Make sure the plate lines up with the bolt; you must be accurate.
5. Mark the holes and pre-drill.
6. Attach the locking plate.

Chain Door Guards

These are installed in a similar fashion as surface bolts, but require much less accuracy. They are installed horizontally on your door.

1. Determine the position of the chain guard.
2. Mark your holes and pre-drill the holes.
3. Attach the chain using the screws provided.

Flip Locks

Flip locks will work only on doors that open toward you. Make sure that you have enough space between the door and door jamb. About $1/8"$ is required so the door will still close after the lock has been installed.

1. Determine the positioning of the lock.
2. Mark the holes and pre-drill.
3. Attach with the screws provided.
4. Close the door and engage the lock.

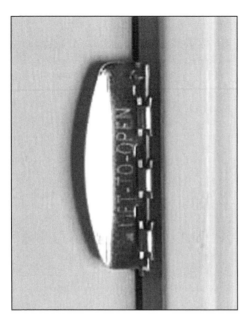

Example of a flip lock.
U 9887 "flip lock" brass plated steel, provided by Prime Line

Top-of-Door Locks

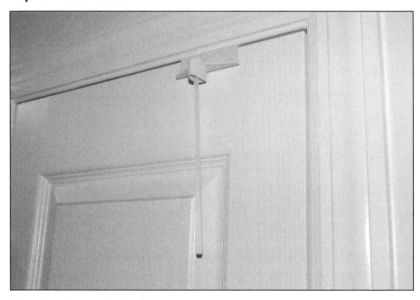

Example of a top-of-door lock.

This lock can be unlocked from either side of the door, which is extremely convenient.

1. Place the locking sleeve on top of the door in the proper direction.
2. Drop in the extender wand.
3. Measure 6" off the door jamb on the header.
4. Mark the hole and make sure that the hole lines up with the sleeve.
5. Pre-drill the hole.
6. Attach the screw in the plastic sleeve provided into the header.
7. Lock the door.

Swing doors are dangerous to have in your house. Not only can little fingers get pinched, but a sibling can get hit in the face (unintentionally, of course!) when standing too close on the other side. These doors should be removed and stored until children are older, secured in a closed position with a surface bolt, or secured in the open position with a door positioner (which sleeves under the door to stop toddlers from swinging it closed).

Bi-fold Locks

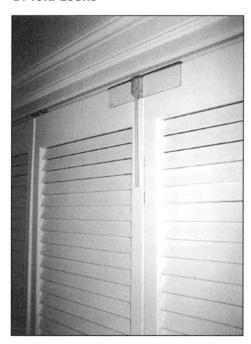

Example of a bi-fold door lock.
Photo courtesy of KidCo, Inc.

These types of locks require a specific amount of space between the top of the door and the track.

1. Place the sleeve over the top of the door and over the fold in the door. This prevents the door from opening.
2. Slide the lock out of the way to open the door.
3. If this lock doesn't work, you can use a shutter bar lock and mount it on the front of the door.

Shutter Bars

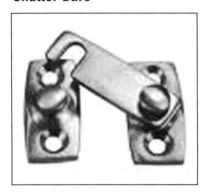

Example of a shutter bar.
Photo courtesy of HandleSets.com

If you have shutters, you'll need this type of lock.

1. Determine the positioning of the lock.
2. Hold the two parts of the lock together over the door fold and mark the holes.
3. Pre-drill the holes.
4. Attach the parts with the screws provided.
5. Engage the lock.
6. Accordion doors and pocket doors can be secured in the open or hidden position. You can also install a pocket door jamb bolt on a pocket door to lock it when it is closed. This requires you to mortise in the lock so the door will still travel in its pocket.

Pocket Door Bolts

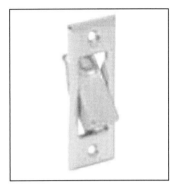

Example of a pocket door bolt.
Photo courtesy of HandleSets.com

Use this lock on a pocket door.

1. Slide out the pocket door.
2. Place the template provided on the door, on the side that goes into the wall.
3. Mark the holes and drill. ***Important reminder:*** You are drilling only partway through the door!
4. Chisel out the wood between the two holes.
5. Pre-dill the screw holes.
6. Attach the bolt using the screws provided.

The most important thing is to create layers of safety. Regardless of whether you install a lock on your interior doors, it's also good to have door knob covers. These are covers that fit over round knobs and require an adult to squeeze two tabs to grab the knob in order to open the door. I don't recommend these as the only safety item to prevent toddlers from gaining access to a room because little fingers do figure out how to work these over time.

Lever handles are the easiest for young children to open. There are several lever handle locks on the market, but most are ineffective. It's best to secure a door with a lever handle in another fashion or replace the lever with a round knob.

Electrical Cords

Electrical cords are dangerous for several reasons: they pose a strangulation hazard if a toddler were to loop one around her neck, they can cause an electrical shock if a toddler (or your pet) were to chew on it, and heavy objects such as lamps can come down on your child's head if they pull on the cord.

Electrical cords can be secured in a variety of ways. Whenever possible, cords should be hidden behind furniture. If that's not an option, you can secure them to the underside of a table or the back of a cabinet using small clamps. You can also use zip ties to secure them to a piece of furniture, such as a table leg. If there are several cords together, they can be placed in a cord cover, which can be attached to the baseboard using adhesive.

Be particularly mindful of cords on items in the nursery, such as humidifiers and baby monitors, because they pose a serious strangulation hazard, as well as the potential of a burn injury should a warm mist humidifier topple down on the baby.

Furniture Strapping and Bracing

Perhaps the safety precaution most often overlooked by families is securing furniture to the wall. Most parents don't think that their toddler has sufficient strength to pull a piece of furniture or a TV down. Sadly, this isn't the case. According to a report by the Consumer Product Safety Commission, in 2006 there were an estimated 42,700 injuries treated at emergency rooms due to topple-over accidents and a total of 180 reported fatalities between 2000 and 2006. Eighty percent of the fatalities were in children under the age of 10, with the ages of 1 to 3 being the most common for injury and death.

Dressers and other items that are small but heavy can become unstable if a child stands on the bottom drawer. I recall reading the tragic story of a mother who lost her three-year-old daughter after a dresser fell on top of her. It was the middle of the night, and there was no sound as the dresser came down on her, killing her within minutes. While the family had secured other heavy furniture to the walls, sadly, the dresser, which seemed strong and stable, was not one of them.

Securing furniture to the wall is inexpensive, easy, and can save lives. Furniture can be secured to walls in two ways, either by strapping or bracing. Furniture strapping is for pieces that are wider than they are tall such as dressers and changing tables. If the piece starts to tip, the straps will go taut to prevent it from toppling over. Furniture bracing is for heavier items to prevent them from moving at all.

Installation How-To's

Furniture Straps (Two Straps per Object)

1. Mark the location of the furniture sides and top.
2. Move the furniture.

3. Locate the studs on the wall using a stud finder. If studs cannot be located, a toggle bolt must be used. If the wall is plaster and lathe studs might be difficult to find, use toggle bolts. If you have a concrete or brick wall, use the appropriate fasteners.

4. Determine the height of furniture when it's against the wall.

5. Measure down 12" to 16" from the top of the furniture height on the wall.

6. Secure the wall side of the furniture strap to the wall.

7. Measure the same distance on the back of the furniture piece.

8. Attach the strap on the back of the furniture using the screws provided.

9. Move the piece back into place.

10. Connect the straps together.

11. Tighten the straps.

Furniture Bracing

You can choose to mount a piece of wood between the wall and furniture or mount an L-bracket to the wall and to the top of the furniture.

Wood Rail Install

1. Mark the location of the furniture sides and top.

2. Measure the distance between the furniture and wall.

3. Move the furniture.

4. Cut the wood rail to the proper length and thickness.

5. Find the studs using a stud finder. If studs cannot be located, a toggle bolt must be used. If the wall is plaster and lathe studs will be difficult to find, use toggle bolts. If you have a concrete or brick wall, use the appropriate fasteners.

6. Attach wood to wall just under furniture height.

7. Move the furniture back into place.

8. Level the furniture.

9. Drill the holes through the furniture into the wood rail.

10. Attach with the screws.

L-Bracket Install

1. Mark the location of the furniture sides and top.

2. Measure the distance between the furniture and wall.

3. Locate the studs on the wall using a stud finder. If studs cannot be located, a toggle bolt must be used. If the wall is plaster and lathe studs might be difficult to find, use toggle bolts. If you have a concrete or brick wall, use the appropriate fasteners.

4. Place the appropriate length L-bracket on top of the furniture against the wall.

5. Attach the L-bracket to the wall.

6. Attach the L-bracket to the top of the furniture to ensure that the screws don't come through the furniture top.

Each child reaches physical milestones at various times, and you cannot determine how quickly *your* baby will be crawling or walking by when other children—even siblings—started doing those same things. Be aware of what your child is doing and anticipate what the next step might be. When considering babyproofing products, such as door locks, gates, and window guards, think of products that take two hands to manipulate which is more difficult for a child.

But you also want to be sure that these products are easy for you to use. Keep in mind that, while they may seem excessive and unattractive, they're intended to be used for a relatively short amount of time while your child is small and inquisitive about everything in the home. It's your job as a parent or caregiver to provide as safe an environment as possible for your child to explore and thrive. So whether you install these products yourself or hire a professional babyproofer, make sure that it's done and done properly. A few nail holes in your walls is a small price to pay for your baby's safety.

Chapter 5

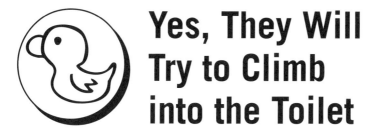

Yes, They Will Try to Climb into the Toilet

I'm often asked which room in the home is most dangerous for kids. Without a doubt, the kitchen and bathroom tie for that distinction. While most people might guess these two rooms, they usually don't realize just how many dangers lurk in these areas.

Please Hold for the Next Operator

You Can't Make This Up

Standing at the sink washing dishes while grilled cheese sandwiches cook on the stove for lunch, I hear a "glug-glugglug" sound behind me. I turn around to find the Nut sitting in front of the open refrigerator with an almost empty bottle of Gaviscon in his hands, the cap sitting next to him on the floor, his lips white with mint-flavored extra-strength antacid. I grab him and smell his breath, as though this will somehow tell me how much he drank. All I learn is that his breath is minty fresh.

Alarmed, but suppressing panic, I call my husband, Jack, to ask him if he remembers how much was left in the bottle. Jack is in the studio rehearsing with a beautiful singer whose name I can't spell, and he doesn't pick up his cell. Pissed off that Jack is probably flirting with a sexy, talented, childless woman while he ignores his phone, I consider the little bottle of Ipecac in the cupboard. Two teaspoons and the Nut'll vomit up everything he's eaten since he was born. Do I really want to put him through that if I don't have to?

I decide to call the emergency room of the local hospital. I look in the phone book, where I happen to find an 800 number for Poison Control. Great idea! The number for Poison Control has been *disconnected!* I call information to see if there's a new number for Poison Control and find myself thinking that James Earl Jones is despicably calm.

Yes, there is a new number for Poison Control. A mellow but attentive woman answers. I am rattled, but manage to read her the ingredients on the Gaviscon bottle in a worried but jaunty manner, hoping maybe she'll be cheerful in return and that my inability to keep my son from drinking things that should be under lock and key eight feet off the ground will be forgiven. She appears to have no sense of humor, but asks me how much he drank.

I hazard a wild guess of four ounces or half the bottle. She puts me on hold! After what seems like eight years, she returns and tells me that he'll probably experience some diarrhea, and I should give him lots of fluids, but

(continued)

that otherwise he should be fine. Relieved, I thank her and hang up, but not before she gets my name, his name, and our phone number, presumably so they can start a folder for me in the Bad Parent File. Oh, the shame! I take a moment just to sit and hug the Nut, who seems fine and not at all poisoned.

Suddenly, I smell something burning. Is it coming from downstairs? Next door? Should I call the fire department? Aaahh! The grilled cheese sandwiches! Turns out there was only a thimbleful of stuff left in the bottle—Jack just hadn't gotten around to throwing it out. And in a matter of hours, it all became an amusing anecdote.

Moral of Today's Story: Put all your emergency numbers by the phone after making sure they're not disconnected. And...everything is always your husband's fault.

Eden Kennedy, founder of fussy.org

Kitchen

For anyone who's ever tried to cook with a toddler underfoot, you know it's not easy. Either they're hanging on your leg or lying in the middle of the floor. Of course, there are also those days when they pull open the drawer, and you walk right into it, trying to suppress the cursing as you watch the bruise on your shin immediately form.

Not only are there sharp objects and hot surfaces in the kitchen, but choking hazards and potentially toxic cleaning products lurk there as well. But the reality is, unless you have a close personal relationship with your pizza delivery guy, you spend a great deal of time in the kitchen, so safeguarding it for your inquisitive toddler is going to be a top priority.

Set Up a Safe Area in the Kitchen

The most important thing is to set up an area where you can see your children, but they are out of harm's way. The area between the stove and the sink is particularly dangerous. Boiling water that you are carrying from the stove to the sink, if spilled on your child, can cause severe burns, usually second degree but occasionally third degree. If possible, set up a play yard in the kitchen or adjoining room where your child is always within sight.

As he gets older, however, and a play yard is no longer an option, it's time to "batten down the hatches." This means securing all the cabinets and drawers with dangerous items such as knives or other sharp utensils or gadgets, cleaning products, and even cooking items like spices, cooking wines, and oils. A good way to keep your toddler occupied is to leave one drawer unlocked for her to play with things such as Tupperware, wooden spoons, and other safe items. If you're worried about her slamming the drawer closed on her finger, you can install two small pieces of wood on the inside of the drawer so it won't shut completely.

Toddlers will become like an eight-armed octopus and reach farther onto a counter top than you would imagine. Keep kitchen cabinets clear of all sharp items, such as knife blocks, and push appliances with cords—toasters, coffee makers, blenders, and food processors—as far back as possible. Cords should be tucked up and out of the way, and be sure to remove from the kitchen anything that your child could step on to gain access to the counter top.

Often, parents overlook the small, seemingly harmless things. One, in particular, is the refrigerator magnet. Ceramic and plastic magnets can fall and break, causing a choking hazard. Several years ago I was filming a TV segment at a family's home. The woman was adamant that her magnets were up high enough on the refrigerator so that her daughter could never pull them off. As the cameras were rolling and we were chatting, she closed the freezer door and, sure enough, one magnet fell off and broke into four pieces, which her toddler immediately picked up.

Lock Down Appliances

Toddlers will imitate their parents, and when they see us going into the refrigerator and grabbing something, they will try to do so also. You'll be shocked the first time you see your little one open the door, reach in, and grab a soda. But, while this may seem cute or funny the first time, there are a host of choking potentials as well as toxic items in a refrigerator. If your child seems to be the type who is drawn to the refrigerator, you may want to consider a refrigerator lock. (This will also help if you've put your hubby on a diet!) Many newer model refrigerators have extremely good seals, but an adhesive mount appliance lock can be used as an extra precaution.

Garbage cans can also contain a host of hazardous items from sharp cans and toxic substances to choking hazards and allergens. They should be kept in a locked cabinet, or you can purchase one that has a heavy lid that is difficult to open. Water coolers should be removed, as they are not extremely stable and can topple over. If it needs to be placed in an area accessible to children, however, it can be secured to the wall with a strap or zip tie. Most water coolers have safety handles for the hot water tap, but they can also be disconnected in the back.

Even washers and dryers should be locked, particularly if they are front loading, as toddlers can get into anything. Sometimes, these machines come with built-in special locking mechanisms, but you can also buy locks online.

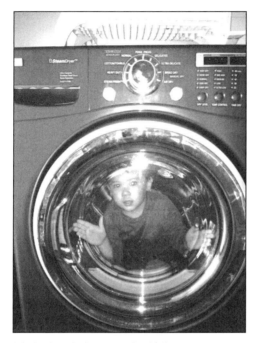

Wash the clothes, not the kid!

If possible, create an area outside of the kitchen to which your children don't have access, to feed your pets. If this isn't possible, keep a close eye on your child as your pet is eating and pick up the animal's food bowls immediately. Pet food should be stored in a locked cabinet or pantry. Water bowls (if they need to be left in the open) should not be breakable. Keep a little water in the bowl and refill often to avoid big spills.

Of course, one of the most dangerous appliances in the kitchen is the stove. Whether burns are caused by reaching up and touching the burner or pulling down a pot, burns from stoves and scalding foods and liquids that spill cause numerous injuries to children. Whenever possible, cook on rear burners and keep pot handles turned toward the back. Stove knob guards can prevent toddlers from turning on the oven and the burners, although they do not fit on the knobs for the newer professional oven brands, such as Viking or Wolf. The knobs for those oven brands can be removed and kept on the counter out of reach of little ones.

Stove guards and stove shields work to prevent toddlers from reaching up to the top of the stove. Stove shields cover only the front of the stove, whereas stove guards also protect the sides of the stove. The issue with these items is they can be difficult to clean, and many people find it inconvenient to cook with them on.

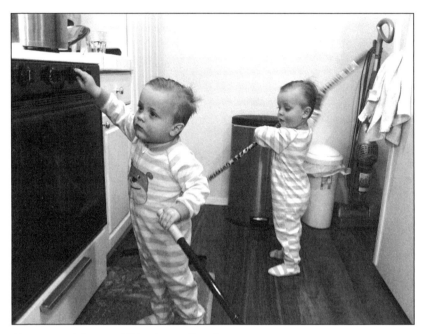

Never, ever let your child get near the stove.

Installation How-To's

＊ Clean your stove surface so it is free of grease.

＊ Attach adhesive clips to the stovetop.

＊ Snap guard/shield into clips.

It's not just burns from touching the hot burner or scalding liquid that are of concern.

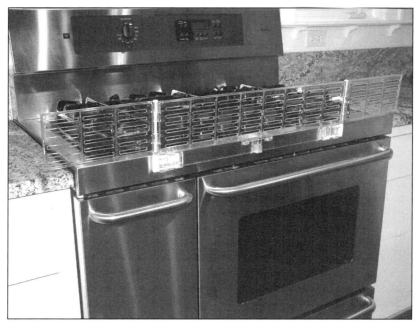

A stove shield protects the front of the stove.

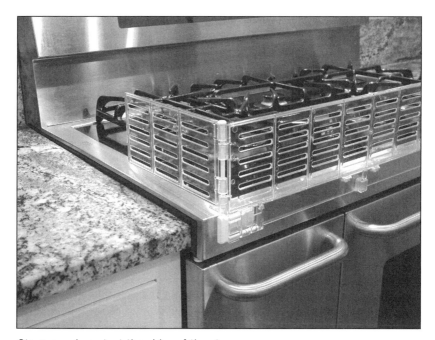

Stove guards protect the sides of the stove.

DID YOU KNOW? DID YOU KNOW? DID YOU KNOW? DID YO

Cooking Fire Hazards

According to the NFPA (National Fire Protection Agency), unattended cooking is the number one cause of house fires, and more than half of home cooking injuries occurred when people tried to fight the fire themselves.

Even the most attentive person will find that, once a baby comes along, it's almost impossible not to become distracted. Sleep deprivation certainly doesn't help. Frying is one of the leading causes of cooking fires. It usually involves hot oil or grease and an open pan. If a frying pan catches on fire, never attempt to use water to extinguish it because it can actually make the fire spread. Even a fire extinguisher, if not used properly, could cause the fire to spread. The best way to attempt to control a frying pan fire is to cover it with a lid.

Despite the fact that fire extinguishers are not appropriate for controlling a frying pan fire, you should always have one nearby and available for other types of kitchen fires, such as when curtains or towels catch fire, or a fire begins in the stove.

While ovens are not as dangerous, they should still be protected with oven locks. They can be installed with heavy duty adhesive and are heat resistant. Some newer models come with built-in locks. Oven locks can also be used for dishwashers. Don't use the handle of the oven as a towel rack. A child could grab onto the towel and try to pull it down, resulting in the oven door coming down on his head.

Cooking with Kids

Even toddlers will enjoy helping out in the kitchen. Cooking with Mom or Dad is a great opportunity for preschoolers to learn about healthy and nutritious foods. Their ability to help out, however, is limited, so find tasks that are age appropriate and safe. Tearing lettuce leaves for a salad, stirring brownie batter, shaping meatballs, and pouring water into a mixing bowl are great jobs for little ones. Be mindful of foods that are choking hazards, such as grapes, raw carrots, and nuts that might be nearby and enticing to them. Set up a prep area for them away from sharp knives, the stovetop, and other electrical appliances. Again, always stress good hand washing after touching any food to avoid cross contamination.

When cooking with siblings of different ages, it's best to have them take turns helping so that you can maintain your complete attention on each one. While an older child is helping cut or stir, a younger brother or sister could be setting the table. When working with your preschooler, an older sibling could read the recipe or write out the menu. Keep your eye on your child at all times. Don't allow yourself to be distracted by another child, the phone ringing, or a delivery person. If you need to walk away, make sure that your child leaves the cooking area as well.

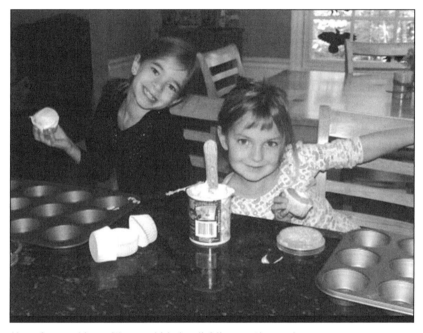

Have fun cooking with your kids by dividing up the work.

Have emergency numbers for the fire department, poison control, and the pediatrician posted on your refrigerator for easy access. Review with your children what they should do if a fire occurs while they're cooking. Make sure they understand that they should not attempt to put it out themselves, but rather get away from the area and follow the pre-designated fire escape plan. Make sure that you are familiar with how to treat various burns, including those from steam, hot grease, and an open flame.

Bathrooms

Bathrooms rank right up there with kitchens when it comes to potential dangers. Drowning, burning, poisoning, deadly falls—all of these accidents can happen in the bathroom. The most important thing to keep in mind is never to leave your child unattended in the bathroom! Whether you have to answer the phone, check on another child, or let the dog back in the house, take your toddler with you. Your baby will not catch a cold from being wet and cold, and a little bit of dripping water on the floor can be wiped up. Sadly, more than 100 children under the age of five die each year from bathtub drownings. Many of these drownings occur when the parents mistakenly believe they have put safeguards in place. It's important to remember that babies can drown in as little as two inches of water.

In some cases, parents may be tempted to leave the bathroom with the water running but the drain open, assuming that the water will drain safely. For various reasons, however, drains can back up, and it takes very little time for the water to rise. In other instances, parents will leave their baby in the tub and put an older sibling in charge. This is just something you can't risk.

Of course, bathtubs are not the only drowning hazard. Yes, kids will fall into toilets, and yes, they can drown. In fact, according to the Consumer Product Safety Commission, over a three-year period, approximately 16 children have died by drowning in toilets. There are some good toilet locks on the market, but one in particular that we like to use at Safety Mom Solutions is the KidCo toilet lock. This lid requires two-handed operation and immediately locks when you close the lid.

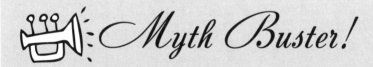

The Real Germy Places in a Bathroom

Myth: You can get an STD (sexually transmitted disease) by sitting on a toilet seat.

According to doctors, this isn't possible. Disease-causing organisms can survive for only a short time on the surface of the toilet seat. Germs would have to travel through a cut or sore to cause infections, which is not likely. In fact, the toilet seat is not even the dirtiest area in the bathroom. The floor, sink, and countertops carry far more germs, which is why it's important to use a paper towel to shut off the faucet once you wash your hands.

Many people think grab bars in a tub are only for seniors, but a surprising number of children are treated in emergency rooms for bathtub falls. In fact, a recent study found that more than 120 children visit the ER on a daily basis for slips and falls in showers and tubs. Most of these children are under four years of age. Grab bars should be installed in all bathtubs and slip-resistant mats placed both inside and outside the tub. Install a tub spout cover to prevent head bumps caused by the faucet.

Burns from hot water are quite common among kids. If you have access to your hot water heater, make sure the temperature is turned down to 120 degrees to prevent scalds. At water temperatures of 125 degrees, a child could receive a second- or third-degree burn after being exposed for just two minutes. If you don't have access to your hot water heater or for added protection, you can install an anti-scald device on your faucets. There are various models that work in different ways, from thermostatically controlled valves to pressure-balanced valves. Decide on the type that's best for you.

You can also purchase one of the bath products that changes color when the water is too hot, but this should never be used exclusively.

When parents think of poisoning, they usually think of the kitchen as the place with toxic cleaning products, but the bathroom has equally dangerous items. Mouthwash, hair gels, and cleansers can all prove toxic to toddlers when ingested. Cabinets and drawers should be locked. Medicine cabinets are particularly important to lock. You should either replace your existing one with a model that can only be opened with a key, or depending upon the cabinet, you may be able to use a cabinet lock, sliding window lock, or adhesive appliance lock. Trash cans should also be kept locked in a cabinet. When organizing your linen closet, be sure to organize it so that safe items such as towels, tissues, and extra toilet paper are on the lower shelves and toiletries, razor blades, and other dangerous items are stored on the higher shelves.

Be certain any electrical appliances, including hair dryers, flat irons, and curling irons are not kept in the children's bathroom, or if your child uses your bathroom, that these appliances are locked away to prevent electrocution. Outlets in the bathroom should be updated with ground fault interruption (GFI) switches, and all outlets throughout the home but especially in the bathroom should be protected with outlet covers. I'm not a fan of outlet plugs, as it's too easy to forget to put them back in. Rather, I prefer the sliding outlet covers, which automatically cover the outlet when not in use. These replace the existing outlet plate and are quite simple to install. There are two types—Decora and Standard, and it depends on what sort of outlet you have which one you decide to use.

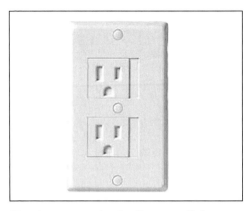

Here is an example of a Decora outlet cover.

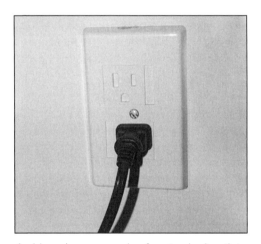

And here is an example of a standard outlet cover.

Home Offices/Gyms/Media Rooms

As someone who works from home, I find it really convenient to be able to multitask: throw in a load of laundry, start dinner, and participate in a conference call at the same time. But arranging things so that my kids understand the boundaries of "mommy's work time" isn't always easy. There's nothing like trying to talk to a client as your kids are screaming about some perceived slight from a sibling. Creating working boundaries is only half the story. Offices were never designed to be child friendly and setting up a home office takes special considerations.

Depending on the location of your home office, establishing a "safe area" within it for your kids to play could be an option. Between computers, printers, fax machines, and other office equipment, wires may be everywhere. This could lead to tripping accidents and electrical hazards. Gather all wires together with wire ties, hide them behind furniture, and cover them with a cord cover.

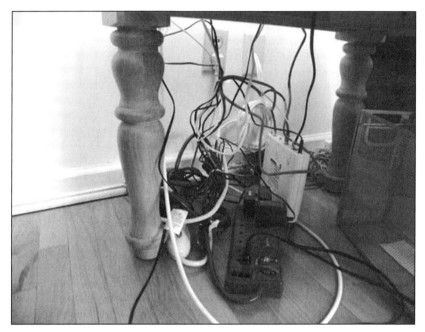

Wires should be tied together and attached to a wall.

Similar to the precautions for other rooms, secure all heavy furniture to the wall and remove any heavy or breakable objects from the tops of tables. Be particularly careful with floor lamps because they can topple over, and get rid of any torchere halogen lamps in the home. Halogen lamps are extremely combustible, and if they touch carpeting, draperies, or fabric on furniture, they will ignite immediately. Office supplies such as staplers, scissors, and sharp letter openers should be kept in a locked drawer. Be sure any throw rugs have a slip-resistant mat underneath them and place foam guards on the corners of any sharp furniture. To prevent embarrassing encounters between your toddler and a client, be sure your email account is not open if you walk away, and teach your child never to pick up your business phone line.

Media rooms have similar issues to those of a home office, but there are other considerations for this room as well. Be sure that you secure the TV to the unit in which it's housed and consider purchasing a faceplate to cover the front of the DVD/VCR player.

Home gyms are extremely dangerous for kids, and children should be kept out of them at all times. Doctors estimate that 25,000 children are treated in emergency rooms annually for home exercise equipment injuries. In 2009, heavy-weight champion Mike Tyson's four-year-old daughter tragically died when she was strangled by the power cable of a treadmill machine. Accidents on treadmills range from burns and lacerations to strangulation. Children will be tempted to come up behind a parent and put their hand underneath a treadmill as it is running. Never leave kids unattended near home exercise equipment, and always be sure to unplug it when you're done. Free weights, jump ropes, and exercise balls should be kept in a locked closet.

Outdoor Areas

If you live in an apartment with an outdoor terrace, remove all furniture or items that your child could stand on and potentially fall over the railing. Be sure that rails on the deck are no more than 2 ⅜" apart. If they are spaced farther than that, you will need to cover the area with a deck railing guard to protect the area. This guard may be fabricated from mesh or other material and attached directly to the railings.

Be sure to keep the terrace door locked at all times and put an alarm on the door so you are alerted when it is opened. The same precautions should be put in place for decks, but also install a gate at the top of the stairs that only opens away from the stairs, not over them. Check each year for wear and tear to the deck—loose nails, splinters, and so on—as well as bees' nests that could form underneath the railings. Secure any free-standing umbrella or patio heater and never leave a child unattended around a heater.

Barbeques on terraces, decks, or patios need to be carefully supervised. Never keep sharp cooking tools dangling from the grill and install a baby gate around the entire perimeter of the grill. If you have plants on the patio and use fertilizer or other chemicals, read the instructions carefully on the packaging and keep children away for a safe period of time. If gardening tools, potting soil, fertilizer, and other similar products are stored in the patio/terrace area, keep them in a locked cabinet.

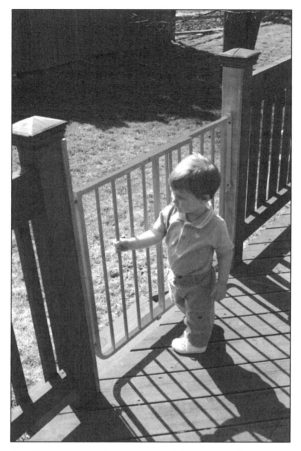

Whether your outdoor area consists of a small patio or
a sprawling backyard, you need to consider some
serious dangers that could harm your little ones.

Garages contain numerous hazards, including power tools, chemicals, and
heavy objects. They should be considered off-limit areas for children, and
any door leading to a garage should have an automatic door closer in addition to a lock. All dangerous items should be placed in locked cabinets in
the garage and other items high up on shelves. Be sure that lawn mowers
are never accessible to children, and when you are mowing, be sure that
kids remain a good distance away from the area.

Back-over Accidents

Without a doubt, though, the most dangerous item in the garage is your car. Back-over accidents are a devastating tragedy and sadly happen all too frequently.

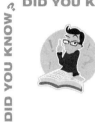

The Rate of Back-over Accidents

Every week at least 2 children are killed and another 50 are injured in back-over accidents. Seventy percent of these happen with a parent or relative behind the wheel. A majority of these involve an SUV or other large vehicle.

You can never assume that your child is safely indoors because they can wander outside without telling you. Install a backup camera in your car and always pull out extremely slowly, stopping occasionally to look around. We're all busy, and it often seems as if we're late for one activity or another. But if you stop and ask yourself whether arriving on time takes precedence over your child's safety, you'll quickly slow down.

The driveway needs to be kept safe as well. Make sure that children understand the boundaries of where they are allowed to play. Keep this area well away from the driveway and preferably out of view from the road. Setting up bright orange cones or some other visual cue will help children recognize the safe area. Even if you have established safe play zone areas, it's too easy for children to forget and run into the driveway after a ball or other toy. They'll also be playing in the driveway if you have a basketball hoop set up or when they're on their riding toys. Consider purchasing a retractable gate to fit across your driveway, as well as signs warning drivers that children are at play. This area should be free of gardening tools, outdoor electrical cords, lawn mowers, and any other hazardous items.

Play Areas

Swing sets, sandboxes, and other play areas need to be secured similar to public playgrounds. Be sure that any play area is visible from the house and check for bees' nests, tree roots, and areas where the ground might have become uneven over the winter as these could all pose risks. Cover sandboxes at night to prevent animals from getting in. Teach your children always to clean up their outdoor toys to prevent an accident with a lawn mower running over them or someone tripping on them.

Pools and Hot Tubs

Pools and hot tubs are the most dangerous areas outside of the home. Drowning is the second leading cause of unintentional injury for kids ages 1 through 14. If you're considering putting in a pool or buying a home with a pool, think carefully. Not only are there significant risks for your own family with a pool, but you also immediately take on the liability if something happens to someone else in your pool.

Many people mistakenly assume that if their children are older and good swimmers, they can rest easy, but sadly many teens drown in pools after drinking, getting injured, or taking risks above their ability. In fact, having a swimming pool can increase your homeowner's insurance premiums dramatically. Regardless of whether you have toddlers or teens, it's imperative that you make your swimming pool or hot tub as safe as possible. A fence should be installed completely around the entire perimeter. A fence that simply surrounds the deck or backyard is not close enough to protect the pool.

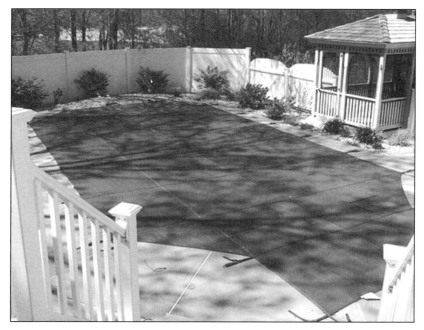

Any pool should be completely surrounded by a fence with a self-latching/closing gate.

Making Your Pool Safe

Four-side fencing completely surrounding a pool could prevent 50–90 percent of accidents.

The fence should not have any foot or handholds, nor should there be any objects such as lawn chairs or riding toys around the fence that your child could use as leverage to climb over. The fence should have a self-closing/self-latching gate as well. If your house opens right onto the pool, the doors leading from the house to the pool should be protected with an alarm. A power safety cover should also be installed. Be sure this cover meets the requirements of the American Society for Testing and Materials (ASTM) pool cover standard that addresses labeling requirements and performance.

If you have an above-ground pool, the steps and ladders leading to the pool should be secured and locked or removed when the pool is not in use. Make sure that there are no toys near the pool, which could entice your child to jump in.

If your child is missing from the house, you should check the pool immediately! Seconds could make a difference between life and death. In a majority of child drownings, the child had last been seen within five minutes. And, unlike the way drownings are portrayed in the movies, they are silent, and you will not hear your child drowning.

It's imperative that you keep a close eye on your child when they are out by a pool. This goes for school-age children and toddlers. Keep a cordless phone at the pool at all times and never leave the kids alone. If you need to go inside to make lunch, or for any other reason, take the kids inside with you. It might seem like a hassle and they might fuss, but it's seemingly brief times like this when accidents occur. If you are having a pool party and inviting additional children to your house, consider hiring a lifeguard to supervise.

Your kids can't live in a bubble, but taking basic precautions will go a long way toward keeping them safe. Whether it's in the kitchen, bathroom, or outside area, be as proactive as possible in preventing injuries. Accidents happen in a matter of seconds and usually are caused by something you've noticed but put off fixing.

Chapter 6

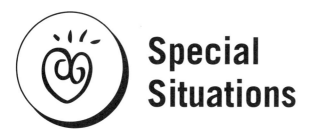

Special Situations

This is without a doubt the toughest chapter for me to write because it's so personal. I'd like to think it can be as irreverent in tone as the rest of the book, but it's impossible. This is about those situations that fall out of the realm of what is considered "normal." The ones that, as parents, can make our hearts break—when we know our children could face insurmountable obstacles as they grow up. This is about our children with special needs and what we need to do to protect them and help them to reach their potential.

My Story

My son Spencer is a strapping, handsome, sweet 12-year-old boy. He has severe intellectual disabilities. His diagnosis is what I like to call "alphabet soup"—ADHD, NVLD, Speech/Language, and Psychosis non-specified. This diagnosis was a long time in coming and took persistence, patience, and a ton of emotional energy to get to it.

When Spencer was born, he was a healthy, happy, and extremely easy-going baby. He was born less than a year after my first son died from SIDS, and it was, to say the least, an extremely emotional time. While everything seemed fine at first, I started to notice things fairly early on. As young as age two, he wasn't interacting with other children in the same way. He crawled late and walked late. But my pediatrician assured me that, while he was a little late developmentally, he still fell within the range of normal. When he turned three and started attending a new day care, the director suggested I see a speech pathologist.

By now, I definitely felt in my gut that something was wrong, but it seemed as if I was the only one who felt that way. Both my mother and Spencer's dad dismissed my concerns. Still, I took him to the speech pathologist. It wasn't until Spencer entered kindergarten that I received more confirmation that indeed Spencer had some "learning disabilities." He was provided with services in his public school, occupational therapy, and speech therapy. This was all new to me, and I was relying on "the professionals" to guide me along. By the time Spencer entered third grade, it was abundantly apparent to me that Spencer had significant issues, although no one could give me a diagnosis. I entered the world of special education and learned phrases such as PPT and IEP. While at the time I was a successful businesswoman, I was as naïve as could be when it came to navigating the political waters of special-ed within the public school system. Whatever I was told, I believed. But still, I knew I had to try and start finding answers why my little boy was "different."

I started doing research on the Internet and reading whatever I could get my hands on. Whenever I ran across an expert who seemed to describe Spencer's issues, I would immediately make an appointment. I dragged him to a multitude of specialists from neurologist to ENTs to sleep specialists and more speech pathologists. I also had him start seeing a psychologist. Still, no one could give me an answer. By now, my mother had accepted that something wasn't right, and to a lesser degree, his dad. I now know that for many fathers, it is hard to accept that their son has a disability. And so, I navigated these waters pretty much on my own while at the same time I had a miscarriage and another baby.

When Spencer's public school decided to retain him in fourth grade, and he started having increasingly troubling interactions with both students and teachers, I knew he was spiraling down, and I had to do something. By then,

I had connected with other parents in town who had special-ed kids. Sadly, it feels like a bit of an underground community. So many people don't speak of their children's disabilities, but when you find the group, the support is amazing. I started getting a lot smarter about the system and hired a special needs advocate and a private therapist to do testing on Spencer. Two years ago, I managed to get Spencer out of the public school system and into a behavioral day school that has made a tremendous difference.

By no means should you take this as a "happily ever after" phrase. Spencer's cognitive development is extremely low, and I've been told that his case is one of the most complex cases anyone has seen. Being the parent of a child with special needs has been one of the most difficult and challenging experiences of my life. There are countless nights where I cry myself to sleep, and I always wonder if there was something I missed or something I should have done sooner. I worry endlessly as to what the future holds for my son, as well as his sisters who will most likely end up responsible for him. But Spencer has also given me incredible joy and taught me some of my most important life lessons. I knew that my fiancé would make the perfect step-father when he told me how grateful he was for having Spencer in his life and how Spencer had taught him about unconditional love.

When my daughter was five, she began to understand that her brother was "different." One day she came home from school and explained how they had read the story of *The Ugly Duckling*. She told me that she realized her brother was just like that beautiful swan and while some of the kids might not see how wonderful he was, she was proud to have a brother who one day would spread his wings and show everyone "his specialness." I knew then that I would never have to worry about who would take care of my son once I was gone.

There's so much more to my story, but I'll save that for another book. I shared this part to help every parent understand that we never know what curve balls life will throw us and our kids. This chapter needed to be included because too many parents of children with special needs or medical issues feel isolated, scared, and frustrated—and sometimes they choose to live in denial. There is support, and while I don't pretend to know about every situation, I can say that Twitter and blogs have become my lifeline to caring and knowledgeable people who have comforted me when I've been at my lowest. It's impossible for me to cover every intellectual, physical, and medical issue in this chapter, but I do want to shed light on some of the greatest concerns and what we all can do to help. *Alison*

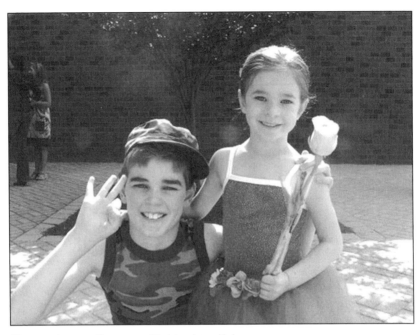

My amazing son Spencer with his sister Kelsey.

Autism

Autism has taken on epidemic proportions. The statistics are absolutely staggering. Prior to 2009, the Centers for Disease Control listed autism as affecting 1 in 150 children, but it is now 1 in 110. Autism affects boys at a much greater rate. In the study conducted prior to 2009, the rate was 1 in 70. With the new statistics, I'm sure it's even higher. The government estimates that the rate of autism is growing 10–17 percent annually! While many parents have heard of autism, unless they have a child with it or know someone who does, they are usually unfamiliar with the symptoms and the challenges that come along with it.

So what exactly is autism? According to Wikipedia "Autism is a highly variable neurodevelopmental disorder that first appears during infancy or childhood, and generally follows a steady course without remission. Overt symptoms gradually begin after the age of six months, become established by age two or three years, and tend to continue through adulthood, although often in more muted form. It is distinguished not by a single symptom, but by a characteristic triad of symptoms: impairments in social interaction; impairments in communication; and restricted interests and repetitive behavior. Other aspects, such as atypical eating, are also common but are not essential for diagnosis."

Symptoms of Autism

There are several different disorders that make up what is considered a part of Autism Spectrum Disorders. These include the following:

* Pervasive Developmental Disorder (PDD)
* Pervasive Developmental Disorder-Not Specified (PDD-NOS)
* Asperger's Syndrome
* Rett Syndrome
* Childhood Disintegrative Disorder

Like me, oftentimes a parent will start realizing that something is not right, but won't be sure exactly what it is. Autistic infants show less attention to social stimuli, smile and look at others less often, and respond less frequently to their own name. You might notice that your child has difficulty making eye contact, difficulty interacting with other children, and difficulty expressing himself or herself. Very rarely will an autistic child initiate play with another child, and they have a hard time with taking turns and responding appropriately to others. For them, reading social cues is close to impossible. The world is very black and white with little room for grays.

Because of this inability, communication becomes challenging. A parent screaming with excitement about some terrific news is no different than a scream of anger or pain for an autistic child. Autistic kids don't understand sarcasm, boredom, or especially teasing. Because of this inability to interact with others, it's extremely difficult for autistic children to form friendships. While autistic children definitely bond with a parent, it doesn't necessarily translate into typical or normal behavior. For example, he may shy away from physical contact, such as cuddling, which is painful for family members and difficult to understand.

Autistic children usually have atypical speech patterns as well, which also makes it challenging for them to convey their emotions. Some will use high-pitched, sing-song voices or flat modulated tones, while others will sound like a "mini-adult" and not understand "kid-speak." This is particularly confusing for family members because they might confuse this mature speaking pattern as just a kid who is extremely mature rather than being autistic.

Autistic kids desperately crave routine and order. They might spend hours lining up toys in a specific manner and need to perform daily routines in exactly the same steps every day. The slightest changes in routine can send an autistic kid over the edge.

Potential Medical Problems and More Symptoms

There are medical symptoms related to autism as well. Many autistic children have gastrointestinal problems (GI), including abdominal pain, chronic constipation or diarrhea, frequent vomiting, and colitis. Studies have shown that nearly 70 percent of autistic children have some sort of GI issue.

Kids with autism have great difficulty in processing and integrating sensory information. They can be overly sensitive to touch, light, sound, smell, taste, and even the movements of others. This is known as Sensory Integration Disorder and can mean that the child is either hyper-sensitive or hypo-sensitive. A child who is hyper-sensitive might have difficulty tolerating the feeling of tags on clothes, zippers on pants, elastic on sleeves, and even certain fabrics. Loud noises from cars or even movies can be disturbing. Attending large parties or merely going to a restaurant with bright lights and loud noises can be particularly difficult for a child on this spectrum. Even small gatherings with several conversations occurring can cause sensory overload and lead to a complete meltdown for an autistic child.

A hypo-sensitive child is just the opposite and has a high threshold for pain. He might require additional stimulus to stay calm, such as eating really crunchy foods or constantly doing jumping jacks, or some other physical activity to keep his body in motion. My son, unfortunately, is both hyper- and hypo-sensitive, which presents a terrific challenge. He literally can't sit still and needs to constantly move around, but loud noises or even several people talking at once will bother him terribly.

Sleep problems are also common in children with autism. Sometimes this is caused by one of the underlying medical issues, such as reflux or sleep apnea, but other times there's no apparent reason. Some researchers think there might be an issue with the regulation of melatonin in autistic kids, but this is just one theory.

Some children with autism have eating disorders in which they will eat non-food items, such as clay, dirt, chalk, and even paint chips. This is known as *Pica*.

While your child's pediatrician should pick up on these cues immediately, it requires parents reporting their concerns in order for a child to be properly diagnosed. So this is where we come to the issue of denial. Because there is still so much mystery surrounding autism, and it's considered to be such a devastating diagnosis for some, many parents will try to ignore the symptoms for a while. Usually, the parent who spends the most time with the child and is witnessing the differences compared to other children will intuitively understand that something is wrong. The other parent or even other family members might convince you that this isn't the case, either because they don't see it as much or choose not to.

Trust Yourself

This is perhaps the most important point I can make in this book: Trust your gut!

You as a parent know your child better than anyone, even medical professionals. Listen to what your inner voice is telling you and keep fighting to find answers and treatment when needed. Do not allow yourself to be dissuaded, even by your pediatrician, when something is wrong with your child. You know what's best for your children, and they will rely on you to protect them and help them. I once received some very sage advice from a friend. In later years, you will always be able to explain to your child why you chose to do something, but never why you chose not to do anything.

While my son has not been given the diagnosis of autism, I see many symptoms of Asperger's in his behavior. If there is a fire drill in school or an assembly that changes his daily routine, he's a mess. He still can't discern when another kid (or even his sisters) is laughing with him or at him. Going to parties and even restaurants can be challenging because it's hard for him to sit still for very long, and interaction with other boys his age is close to impossible.

The greatest challenge arises when a parent does not seek help and learn about dealing with autism. Family arguments can quickly arise when a grandparent or even a spouse who doesn't understand the specifics of autism merely considers your child "out of control" or rude. I've heard numerous stories of families torn apart when autistic children were reprimanded and told to behave and sit down and moms were queried as to why their child wouldn't give hugs. For parents of an autistic child, it's vital to reach out for support within the autism community and learn how to help your child create a safe and successful life.

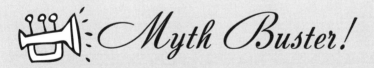

Divorce and Autism

Myth: The rate of divorce among parents of autistic children is 80 percent.

This statistic was debunked in a survey that was conducted in 2010, which showed that couples with an autistic child had a divorce rate of 64 percent while the general population was 65 percent. For couples who did divorce, they noted that their child's autism diagnosis was not the cause, but only one of the contributing factors.

A diagnosis of autism affects the entire family and absolutely adds a level of stress. But for those with a strong foundation, it can actually make a couple closer as they bond together to help their child.

That Feeling of Guilt

Parents always live with guilt and often when there is a diagnosis of autism or some other neurological issue, they will immediately wonder what it was that they did wrong and how they caused it. They literally are desperate to find a cause and ultimately find a cure. I know that feeling only too well. We'll chase any new theory and cure in hopes of helping our child. The unfortunate reality is that no one really understands the cause of Autism Spectrum Disorder (ASD) or why it is increasing so rapidly. For many years, there was a loud group of parents who believed that childhood vaccines caused autism. This was fueled by the claims of a former British surgeon and medical researcher, Dr. Andrew Wakefield, who conducted a study of 12 children in 1998 that showed a connection between the Measles, Mumps, Rubella (MMR) vaccine and autism. Advocates and celebrities alike jumped on this bandwagon and very publicly spoke about the dangers of vaccines. It's important to note that there have been similar claims regarding the link between Sudden Infant Death Syndrome and vaccines as well. In 2010, Dr. Wakefield was found guilty of acting unethically during the time he conducted the study. The United Kingdom's General Medical Council concluded that Wakefield participated in "dishonesty and misleading conduct."

Pediatricians and many autism experts for years have stated that there is no proof of a connection between autism and vaccines. And, in fact, the dangers of not vaccinating your child are far greater. Please understand that I'm not saying that it might not be better to spread the time of the administration of these vaccines out, but it is vital that parents understand the dangers of *not* vaccinating children.

Once you can accept a diagnosis of ASD, the sooner you can begin helping your child and keeping him safe. While many of the safety measures covered in this book will apply, there are additional steps you should take for an autistic child.

Get Support

Perhaps the most important thing is to enlist support for yourself. You will be able to find local support groups in your area, but the Internet is an amazing place to find any information you need. Simply realizing that other people are facing the exact challenges you are facing helps immensely. A great source of information and support is the organization Autism Speaks (*www.autismspeaks.org.*) They can put you in touch with local groups and keep you up-to-date on the latest research. Another great resource is an Internet radio show Coffee Klatch (*www.thecoffeeklatch.com*), which features various guests discussing topics concerning children who have a variety of disabilities both physical and emotional.

It's important to sit anyone down who interacts with your child and explain what autism is and how they can help him feel more comfortable. Many people simply don't understand, so it might also be helpful to point them to specific Web sites and blogs. They need to understand that your child's well-being is the top priority and that there might be occasions where you need to leave a family gathering early or not show up at all if it's a bad day for your child. No matter where you go, accommodations and safety measures must be established, and this might require you and your partner to be less available to socialize in order to watch your child.

All parents, but especially those of a child with special needs, need a break every now and then. Caring for your child can be exhausting and emotionally draining. Once again, a happy mommy is a happy child, and in order to have the patience required to care for your child, you need a break every now and then to recharge yourself. Finding an appropriate caregiver for your child is not easy, however. While some au pair and nanny agencies will advertise that they have specially trained staff to care for children with special needs, this isn't always the case, and the level of care can vary tremendously. Language and cultural miscommunications can occur as well. A young au pair coming over from an Eastern European country might understand the term *special needs* to be quite different than what your situation requires. If your child attends a preschool or some class, you can ask one of his teachers if they babysit. You can also ask friends in the community who have a child with autism if they have a referral, or it might be better to find a top-notch babysitter whom you trust and work with her to teach her specifically how to care for your child. Sometimes, all of the training in the world won't help when it comes to your specific situation.

Childproofing Is a Must

You will have to be hyper-vigilant in babyproofing your home and being sure that wherever you go is safe. Autistic children not only tend to wander, but they are attracted to water. Monitors should be placed on all windows and doors, and you should consider putting a motion detector in your child's room so you will know if he gets up in the middle of the night. Some towns have now created "Autistic Child Area" traffic signs that can be placed in neighborhoods.

Call your local police department and alert them to the fact that you have an autistic child and at the very least they can place "Children at Play" signs there. It's definitely important to alert your local police to the fact that you have an autistic child in case he does wander. You might need to educate them a bit as to his specific issues: Is he verbal? Does he have an aversion to touch? Will he run away from police car lights or sirens? Make sure that your child always has his address and phone number attached to an article of clothing that he's wearing, an ID bracelet, or a chain or tag for his shoe. Make sure that neighbors know that your child is autistic and ask them to always keep their eyes open if they see him wandering. Keep all car doors locked so that he can't get in and potentially lock himself in, especially on a hot day.

Motions detectors and locks on the windows and doors are just a start. Every drawer and cabinet in both the kitchen and bathroom must be locked. Never leave knives or other sharp objects on the kitchen counters. Keep the refrigerator locked to prevent him from getting into food he shouldn't. For children who tend to chew, be careful of all small and even at times large objects because they might put anything in their mouths.

Siblings' toys need to be carefully supervised and locked away when not in use. Items with strings or cords should be avoided since they can become strangulation hazards. All furniture should be secured to the walls, and TVs need to be secured into a cabinet. Electrical outlets should be covered, and cords should be tied to the sides of table legs.

When traveling, keep an ID tag and medical information in the glove box and attached to the side of any car seat. If you are rendered unconscious, emergency workers need to be aware of your child's condition.

I have no idea what the future holds for my son. Every day he leaves for school I worry about his safety and whether he'll be happy. I try to relax, but any parent of a child with special needs knows that we're always on our guard. I do, however, grow increasingly hopeful as I meet more parents online and see that their children have found their own way in the world. I pray this will also be the case for my son.

Cerebral Palsy

I'm amazed at how prevalent premature births are in this country. My cousin's daughter was barely two pounds when she was born, and my friend's twins were born at one pound each.

Rate of Premature Birth in the United States

In the United States, more than half a million babies, or one in every eight, are born premature each year.

Prematurity is the leading cause of death among newborns. For those who survive, they face lifelong medical issues that include cerebral palsy (CP). Approximately 800,000 children and adults in the United States have CP. About 3 in every 1,000 are affected. Children are usually diagnosed by the age of three.

Cerebral palsy refers to a group of conditions that affect movement, balance, and posture. The most common symptoms are a lack of muscle coordination when performing voluntary movements; stiff or tight muscles and exaggerated reflexes; walking with one foot or leg dragging; walking on the toes, a crouched gait, or a "scissored" gait; and muscle tone that is either too stiff or too floppy. Symptoms range from mild to severe, but do not get worse as the child gets older. With treatment, most children can significantly improve their abilities.

Many children with cerebral palsy have other conditions that require treatment. These include mental retardation, learning disabilities, seizures, abnormal physical sensations (difficulties with sense of touch), and problems with vision, hearing, and speech.

Again, it's easy to blame yourself for something that you really had no control over. Allow yourself time to accept the diagnosis, but then get to work helping your child. Physical therapy can begin as soon as a diagnosis is made, but don't push your child beyond his limits. Because his balance and coordination are compromises, be careful of falls. Make sure any rugs in the house have non-skid mats underneath and that there are treads on all staircases. Install a grab bar in the bathroom and be sure that there's always a non-slip mat in the tub. All furniture needs to be secured to the wall to prevent topple-over accidents if he is grabbing on.

Since a child with CP can have difficulty chewing and swallowing, you need to be particularly cautious when feeding him to avoid choking.

The Role of Environmental Toxins

Many people question the role of environmental toxins in many disabilities. Exposure to a number of environmental health hazards during pregnancy has been associated with birth defects, low-weight babies, premature births, or an increased risk of miscarriages. These include various chemicals, such as paints, dry cleaning chemicals, and pesticides, as well as heavy metals like lead, cadmium, and mercury. Many researchers also feel there is a link between environmental toxins and autism, as well as other developmental disorders.

I strongly believe that the cause for the dramatic increase in developmental disabilities must be linked to the growing amount of toxins in our world and the exposure our children are subjected to even before they're born. In July 2005, the Environmental Working Group released results of a study they conducted using cord blood to determine the level of chemical exposure in utero. The findings were disturbing. Of the 287 chemicals identified in the umbilical cord blood of 10 infants, 180 were known carcinogens, 217 were toxic to the brain and nervous system, and 208 have been associated with birth defects or abnormal development in animal tests.

Chemical Toxins

Over the past several years, the Food and Drug Administration (FDA) has been looking into the dangers of the chemicals bisphenol-A (BPA) and phthalates, which are used in hundreds of plastic consumer products to make them hard or flexible. They are used not only in adult consumer products, but also in baby bottles, plastic dishes, and other products our children frequently use. They can also be found in virtually every can of food in the U.S. food supply within the thin plastic liners. When these products are heated up, placed in the dishwasher, or become old, the chemicals can leach into the environment, namely your body. BPAs are a known endocrine disruptor with the potential to disrupt the body's hormone levels and are particularly dangerous for babies and pregnant women. They can affect the neurological development of infants and young children. Because there are so many plastics in our society, nearly every American has some amount of BPA in their body. While the FDA expressed "some concerns" about the potential impact of BPA on the brains of fetuses, infants, and children, they have yet to call for a ban.

Other countries, however, have already led the way. France and Canada recently banned the use of BPA altogether in baby bottles. And while the federal government might be unwilling to act, local and state governments are. Many cities and counties around the country have banned BPAs in baby products. Even retailers such as Walmart and Toys"R"Us no longer carry products containing BPAs. Many baby bottle manufacturers now have BPA-free bottles, and you can research online which ones are safe. Additionally, avoid plastic bottles that have a #3, #5, or #7 on the bottom, as these contain BPAs. It's almost impossible to completely eliminate BPAs from your home because virtually all canned goods have them, but you can minimize your exposure. Also, do your research and write to your local representatives if you live in an area that has not yet banned BPAs.

Phthalates are chemicals that are used to make plastics soft and pliable. They are found in a variety of products including the following:

* Baby toys, teethers, pacifiers

* Cling wrap

* Shower curtains

* Personal care products such as deodorants, nail polishes, perfumes, and cosmetics

* PVC and vinyl flooring

In animal studies, phthalates have been connected to problems with the liver, kidneys, lungs, and reproductive systems. Scientists at government agencies in both the United States and Canada agree that exposure to the chemicals could cause a wide range of health and reproductive problems in people. In a recent study by the Centers for Disease Control, researchers found phthalates in virtually every person tested, but the largest concentrations were found in women of childbearing age, almost 20 times higher than the average population.

In 2009, the findings of a study conducted by Swedish and American scientists were released linking the presence of vinyl flooring (containing phthalates) in a parent's home and autism in their children. The study was based on surveys that asked a variety of questions related to the indoor environment. Of the study's 4,779 children between the ages of 6 and 8, 72 had autism, including 60 boys. The researchers found four environmental factors associated with autism: vinyl flooring, the mother's smoking, family economic problems, and condensation on windows, which indicates poor ventilation. Infants or toddlers who lived in bedrooms with vinyl or PVC floors were twice as likely to have autism five years later, in 2005, than those with wood or linoleum flooring.

While the study is by no means conclusive, it does raise concerns. Pre-term labor, Autism Spectrum Disorders, learning disabilities, and a host of other developmental disorders are being caused by something. Environmental toxins are being pointed at for the cause of a number of medical issues as well. These "environmental illnesses" include symptoms such as nasal congestion, fatigue, headaches, hyperactivity, muscle or joint pain, twitches, blurred vision, burning skin, abdominal discomfort, and the inability to think clearly, as well as a variety of learning or behavior difficulties. Experts acknowledge that, in many instances, childhood leukemia and childhood cancers are not genetic, but actually are triggered by chemicals.

What to Do About Toxins

It's almost impossible to remove all of the environmental toxins from our home, but the more we can do, the better off we'll be. Becoming aware of the problems and some healthier alternatives is the first step.

Clear the Air

My mother always used to throw open the windows to "air out the house" as she said. Turns out she was on to something. Common household cleaners and home improvement items such as wet paint, new carpet, and treated wood, as well as all of those lovely air fresheners we use to make our homes smell lovely, emit fumes that contain chemicals. Without ventilation, they will attach to dust particles on the floor and fibers in fabric, such as carpets, curtains, and upholstery.

Carpet shampoos usually leave a sticky residue on carpet fibers that are usually hard to see or feel. Not only does the residue attract and latch onto dirt but children, who crawl and play on carpets, can inhale them or get them on their hands, which they then put into their mouths.

Powders or dusts are easily inhaled and may irritate airways and cause asthma attacks. In fact, anti-dust-mite carpet treatments sometimes contain tannic acid or benzyl benzoate, both of which are skin, eye, and respiratory irritants. Whether it's dry cleaning, new carpet, or furniture that has been treated with stain repellant, all of these items pose a health hazard due to chemicals. Be sure to remove bags from around dry cleaning items immediately and provide sufficient ventilation for new carpet and stain-treated furniture. The best solution is to open windows and use exhaust fans that will allow the chemicals to escape.

Toss the Cleaners

We've been brainwashed by companies into thinking that, when it comes to cleaning products, stronger is better. This is especially true with the advent of antibacterial soaps, toothpastes, and other personal care products. The reality is that outside the hospital setting antibacterial products are not necessary and, in fact, can be potentially harmful. The active ingredient in antibacterial products is triclosan, which according to the EPA (Environmental Protection Agency), "is suspected to be" contaminated with dioxins, highly carcinogenic chemicals. Household cleaners can also be highly toxic. Mixing an ammonia-based product with chlorine bleach creates poisonous gas.

What's more, the bright colors of some cleaners can be attractive to children. According to the Consumer Products Safety Commission (CPSC), glass cleaners accounted for 9,418 calls to poison-control centers during a recent year. Fortunately, there are many effective and safe alternatives on the market today. For protecting kids from germs, good hand washing is just as effective as antibacterial soaps. Teach kids proper hand washing techniques and make sure they wash often. Wash their toys regularly as well. All natural cleaning products such as vinegar, baking powder, and lemon juice are highly effective in cleaning appliances and surfaces. There are also several great lines of green cleaning products in stores today.

You Are What You Eat

While the EPA is tasked with monitoring the level of pesticides used on food, the level is still too high. Some of the fruits and vegetables with the highest levels of pesticides are the ones that kids love the most—apples, celery, peaches, and pears. Exposure to these pesticides builds up over the years and can cause serious health issues, including developmental delays, behavioral disorders, and motor dysfunction.

Try to select organic produce at your grocery store or shop at local farmer's markets for organic produce. Beware of labels, however! "Natural" does not mean it's organic. In fact, it's an unregulated term that can be placed on any product, which makes it quite misleading. Only the "USDA Organic" label indicates that a food is certified organic.

Get the Lead Out

Another factor that has been linked to autism is lead poisoning. There is no definitive conclusion, but the symptoms of lead poisoning are very similar to traits of autistic children. Lead can be most often found in older homes with chipping paint, but it is also found in a variety of products from construction materials to batteries. Each year in the United States, 310,000 1- to 5-year-old kids are found to have unsafe levels of lead in their blood. Even low levels of lead exposure can cause permanent neurological damage in children including:

* Nervous system and kidney damage
* Learning disabilities, attention deficit disorder, and decreased intelligence
* Speech, language, and behavior problems
* Poor muscle coordination
* Hearing damage

Immediate symptoms can also, like mold exposure, appear like cold and flu symptoms—tiredness, irritability, loss of appetite, difficulty sleeping, and constipation. Babies in the womb who are exposed to lead can experience stunted growth and learning difficulties. When pregnant women are exposed to lead, it can lead to premature birth.

Lead paint in your home is a hazard even if it isn't peeling, chipping, or cracking. It's especially dangerous when it's on high-use surfaces including the following:

* Windows and windowsills
* Doors and doorframes
* Stairs, railings and banisters
* Porches and fences

If your home was constructed prior to 1978, there is a high likelihood that lead-based paint was used. If you think that your child was exposed to lead, your pediatrician can do a simple blood test to determine if she has lead poisoning.

You will then need to test for lead in your home and eliminate it. You can have your home inspected for lead paint, but don't remove it yourself. Sanding down lead paint or removing the paint yourself can release dangerous levels of lead dust. You will need to hire a contractor who's qualified to remove it safely. Have your drinking water tested as well. Lead in drinking water can come from old well water or from old plumbing materials and water service lines.

Probably the most difficult aspect for a parent of a child with special needs is the mystery surrounding a cause. We desperately want something to blame and the magic bullet that will make it all go away. I hope even those of you who do not have a child with special needs have taken the time to read this chapter. It's easy to look away from issues that don't affect us directly and pretend these things don't exist, but as parents we need to support each other and teach our own children tolerance and acceptance.

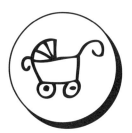

Chapter 7

Taking Baby Out— You Can't Babyproof the World

Often, new parents will get advice from grandparents not to take a newborn outside for the first six weeks. This is one of those bits of wisdom that will be handed down for generations, but it just isn't accurate. Not only do *you* need to get out of the house to prevent yourself from going stir-crazy, but it's also good for your baby to go outside, just in the appropriate places and armed with the necessary supplies.

What you will quickly come to learn is that social boundaries fly out the window once you have a baby. Complete strangers feel entitled to touch your baby and offer unsolicited advice (and they will be insulted if you don't take it!). While the attention your baby receives is nice, it can also lead to a host of germs getting near her, especially in the winter months when more people are indoors at malls and grocery stores sneezing and coughing.

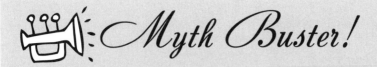

You Don't Get a Cold from the Cold

Myth: Going outside without a hat, coat, gloves, or with wet hair and getting chilled or overheated causes a baby or child to get sick.

Cold germs are caused by viruses. The reason more colds happen in the winter months is because people are generally inside more and in closer proximity to one another. Cold viruses survive longer when the humidity is low, which is the case in the colder months.

What will make your baby sick is contact with someone who is carrying germs. So, most importantly, keep strangers from touching your baby. Be sure that your older children and all other family members frequently wash their hands.

Going Outside

When heading out for the first few weeks with your baby, stick to places that are less populated, and you run less of a risk of strangers touching your baby. This is not to say that when you go somewhere, your baby shouldn't be dressed appropriately. A good rule of thumb is one more layer on your baby than you have on yourself. Whether it's sunny or cloudy, you need to protect your baby from ultraviolet rays.

Babies under six months of age should be kept out of the sun completely. That means using the shade on your stroller and being sure that you have her dressed loosely but in tight-woven fabrics (fabrics that are hard to see through, which will block out the sun's rays).

In the summer, keep a wide-brimmed hat on your baby to protect his face. It's not recommended to use sunblock on babies under six months of age, but if there are a few exposed areas on his body, use only minimal amounts on his face and the back of his hands.

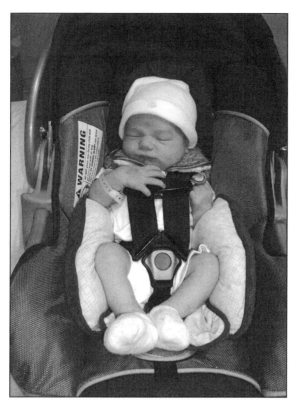

Everyone wants to touch a baby!

Quick strolls after feeding are easy and don't require much thought, but if you plan on being out over an extended period of time, you need to be geared up for the excursion. The first few times trying to remember everything you should take with you is stressful, to say the least. And, invariably, you *will* forget something (sleep deprivation doesn't help). Trying to be prepared for every scenario isn't easy, but if there are a few places you visit frequently, you might want to keep supplies labeled for that destination in a Ziploc bag ready to go. For example, if you live near a beach or belong to a pool club, you might want to keep a bag stocked with sunscreen, a hat, baby wash and shampoo, and some items for yourself in one bag labeled "beach" or "pool." Frequent trips to grandma's house might require you to have some extra toys, blankets, and pacifiers on hand.

But, no matter where you go, a well-stocked diaper bag is essential for surviving an outing with your baby or toddler.

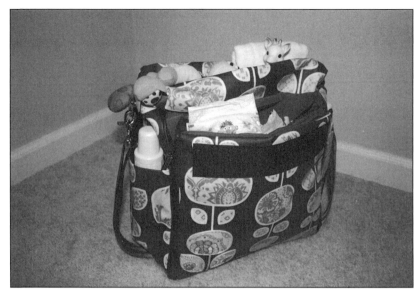

Diaper bags come in all shapes and sizes, but it's what's inside them that counts.

Here's what you'll absolutely need in your bag:

* Two to three extra changes of clothes, including undershirts and socks. Pack an extra shirt for yourself if you need to look good, as chances are your baby will spit up on you!

* Two lightweight blankets

* Extra diapers, at least six or seven

* Wipes

* Two baby toys, teething rings, and a stuffed animal

* Crayons, books, and other toddler toys

* Ziploc bags for soiled items

* Non-alcoholic hand sanitizer gel

* Extra formula and bottles (if you are not nursing) and sippy cups

* Two bottles of water—one for you and one for your baby

* Extra nursing pads if you are nursing

* Diaper rash cream

* A washable mat for changing your baby

* Extra pacifier if your baby uses one

✳ List of emergency information and numbers, including those for poison control, your pediatrician, a secondary emergency contact if something happens to you, medical insurance information, and a list of any medical issues your baby might have.

✳ A nasal syringe, thermometer, and saline spray to clear stuffy little noses and Band-Aids. If you have an older child along with you, pack a first aid ointment such as Neosporin NEO TO GO and an antihistamine, such as Children's Benadryl.

✳ Get one small pack to keep all your items together—cell phone, keys, money, credit cards, lip gloss (you might want to try and keep up appearances), and ID.

✳ If your baby is eating solids, pack a snack pack with Cheerios or some toddler snack.

✳ Disposable place mat, a plate, bowl, and spoon

✳ Baby food in non-breakable jars

In addition to always having your diaper bag on hand, keep a first aid kit in your car. This should contain the same items as your home first aid kit, as well as a blanket, calamine lotion, tweezers, a flashlight, emergency medical information for first responders, a barrier device for CPR, and an antiseptic wash in case you're not near a water source.

One thing many people don't think of is having an extra cell phone in your first aid kit. You don't have to have a contract for this phone; by law, you must be able to dial 911 from it. It needs only enough battery power to make that one phone call. So, if you're upgrading your phone for whatever reason, throw the old phone into your car's first aid kit.

Riding Toy Safety

Every parent thinks about the first tricycle they'll buy their child. The image of him tearing around, pedaling his little feet is the quintessential childhood memory. But whether it's a tricycle, bicycle, "Barbie car," or Razr Scooter, ride-on toys need to be used with caution.

There are tricycles and other ride-on toys that even toddlers can use, but other things, such as scooters and skateboards, shouldn't be used until a child is at least three or four years of age, depending upon his ability. When a kid sees a tricycle under the Christmas tree with a big red bow on it, he's going to be itching to try it out, and if you live in colder climates where riding outside isn't an option, you'll be tempted to let him test out the wheels inside. A child who is just learning to ride isn't going to have the ability to steer and stop properly, and when he is riding inside the house, he runs the risk of losing control and going down a flight of stairs, knocking over a heavy object, or smashing into the side of a table. Keep riding toys for outdoor fun.

From day one, teach your kids the importance of safety gear no matter what riding toy they're using. Nationally, nearly 300,000 children 14 and under are treated in hospital emergency rooms every year for bicycle-related injuries. Almost half of these are diagnosed with a traumatic brain injury.

When worn properly, bicycle helmets have been shown to reduce the risk of head and brain injury by as much as 85 percent. In fact, bike helmets are so important that the U.S. government has established safety standards for them. Your child's bike helmet should have a sticker on it from the Consumer Products Safety Commission (CPSC), which indicates that it has met these safety guidelines. Also be sure that the helmet fits properly. It should be worn level, cover the forehead, and be snug enough that it can't move around on your child's head.

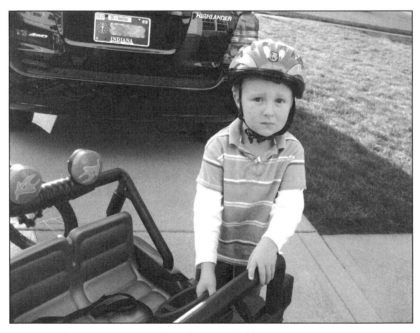

Bicycle helmets save lives—with all kinds of ride-on toys.

In addition to wearing a proper helmet, here are a few more tips to ensure a safe ride:

∗ **Read the manufacturer's instructions.** Be sure that that your child fits the height, weight, and age requirements. Follow assembly instructions carefully and check for any sharp edges, loose parts, or missing screws.

∗ **Check the fit.** Your child should be able to reach the pedals easily while sitting squarely on the seat, and her knees must not hit the handlebars or steering wheel. Make sure the bike has an adjustable seat or frame so you can adjust it as she grows.

∗ **Clear the area.** Make sure that the area he is riding in is free of any obstacles such as twigs, tree stumps, and other toys. Be on the lookout for wet leaves, sand, gravel, storm grates, curbs, and puddles. Clearly set boundaries where it is permissible for your child to ride and post a sign that alerts anyone coming into the driveway that a child is riding.

∗ **Wear the right gear.** Dress your child in bright clothing so that they are easy to see. Check for loose clothing, shoelaces, and backpack straps that could get caught in the wheel. Be sure that they wear sneakers rather than flip flops or cleats, which won't grip the pedal.

∗ **Understand the rules of the road.** If he will be riding in the street, be sure your child understands basic road rules:

  ∗ Learn and use appropriate hand signals

  ∗ Stop and check for traffic both ways before leaving a driveway or entering an intersection

  ∗ Never ride against traffic

  ∗ Use bike lanes or designated bike routes whenever possible

  ∗ Ride single file when riding in the road

  ∗ Stop at all stop signs and obey traffic lights just as a car would do

Surviving the Playground Jungle

I sometimes feel that the playground is rather like the ancient gladiator stadiums. Our kids are thrown in with other kids who are wild and out of control, as clueless babysitters and distracted parents look on. The first time you witness your child being pushed or hit by another child, you will be horrified and want to take the offending little demon and wrap him around the monkey bars. You will be equally horrified when the demon's parent doesn't take notice or worse, does take notice but fails to reprimand him or her. What's a parent to do?

Interacting with Other Children

Obviously the first priority is to make sure that your child isn't hurt and then intercede. Whenever possible, it's best to speak to the bully's parent or caregiver rather than the bully himself. Give that parent or caregiver the benefit of the doubt. She might have been distracted and not noticed the incident. As calmly as possible, speak with the parent and explain what you observed. Ask her to speak with her child and, ideally, all speak together so that the children can be a part of the solution. Unfortunately, things might not go that smoothly. You might get the fallback excuse "kids will be kids" from the parent, or you might be unable to locate the bully's parent.

Then is the time to take matters into your own hands. The bullying may stop after your first intervention, but keep a close eye on your child and the bully. If your child is pushed or hit again, you have every right to step in and protect her. Talk to the bully yourself and let him know that not only is hitting not allowed, but you will both be going over to explain to his caregiver what just happened. If the playground is part of a private club or children's center, immediately alert a staff member. Many of these places have strict policies regarding appropriate behavior, and the offending child and his parents will be prohibited from returning after two or three incidents. I'm happy to say, however, that most parents and caregivers respect the parental code of protecting their young and will cooperate with you in taming their little beast.

So what *do* you do when *your* child is the bully? It's important to first assess the situation and take a time-out with your child. If it's an isolated incident that happened once on the playground, perhaps it's a matter of your child being tired or hungry. But, if there is an ongoing pattern and you're hearing about it not only from playground moms but also preschool teachers, you need to take a careful look at what's going on. Some children have a hard time socializing with other kids and will act out in order to get attention. They might also be witnessing bully behavior from other children. Try to do some role playing with your child or maybe even act out some scenarios with dolls, puppets, or stuffed animals. Be sure they're not witnessing bully-like behavior at home, such as spanking or hitting. The consequences for bullying behavior should never be any sort of physical punishment because this will completely send the wrong message. Drawing a picture for the child that was bullied or taking away some privilege will be more effective.

Checking Out Playground Equipment

Aside from playground bullies, there are other safety concerns to consider at local playgrounds. Every year more than 200,000 kids are injured on playgrounds. A majority of these accidents are due to falls and usually occur on public playgrounds, although nearly 20 percent do occur on home playground equipment.

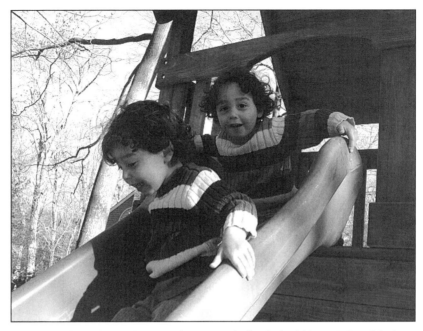

Kids love slides, but make sure they are safe (both the kids and the slides).

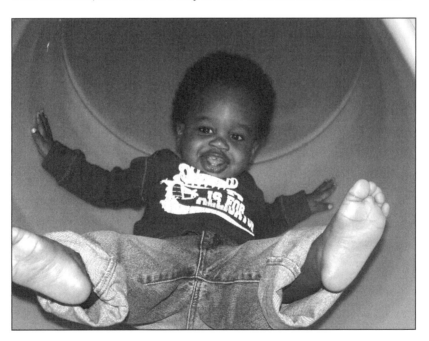

Unfortunately, there are no mandatory state laws for public playgrounds, although the Consumer Product Safety Commission has developed guidelines for both public and home playground equipment. These can be found on the CPSC's Web site. There are some states that have already adopted these guidelines. In order to determine if your state is one of them, you can visit the National Program for Playground Safety (NPPS) Web site (*www.playgroundsafety.org*) and review their state regulations page.

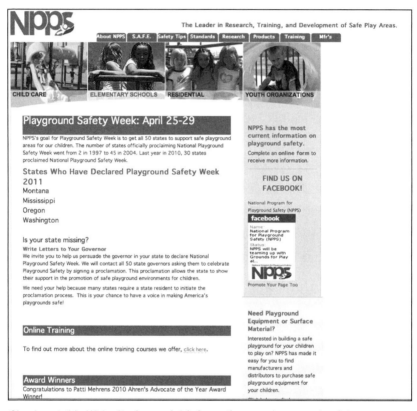

Check out this Web site for useful information on playground safety.

Even with these safeguards in place, it's still ultimately up to parents to check out a playground carefully before allowing their kids to play there. The NPPS also has a "Playground Report Card" that you can download and use to check your local playground. You can review it at *www.playground safety.org/safe/grade_your_own.pdf*.

Here are a few things to consider:

✳ **Is every area of the playground visible?** Will you be able to see your child at all times, or are there trees or other items obstructing certain areas? If your child is seriously hurt, you need to know immediately.

✳ **Does it have a safe ground covering?** Playgrounds should be covered with mulch, rubber shreds, sand, and other loose-fill materials or rubber mats. Grass, cement, asphalt, and dirt are not safe. It's also important to have the appropriate depth for ground covering. It should extend out at least six feet around the entire perimeter of any stationary piece of equipment. For items such as swings, it should be double the swing zone. In other words, if a swing is 10 feet high, the ground covering should extend out 20 feet.

✳ **Is the equipment well maintained?** After years of use and particularly after harsh winters, playground equipment can become rusty or damaged. Push on the stands holding swings and make sure they are still solidly bolted to the surface. Tug on the swing itself and look at the "S" hooks to be sure that the swing is still sturdy and being held in place. Check for any wood surfaces that have splintered or cracked and metal surfaces with rust.

✳ **Is the equipment old?** Standards have changed over the years, and if your playground is old, it might have equipment that is now considered unsafe. There should be no openings on any equipment between 3 ½" and 9", which could cause an entrapment hazard. Of particular concern are the areas at the top of slides and climbing bars, which could have an opening of this size. Also, check for any equipment that might have a "V" opening at the top, which could pose a strangulation hazard.

✳ **Is the playground set up for safety?** A two-year-old's ability is very different from that of a four-year-old. There should be a separate area for younger children with age-appropriate equipment. Also, be sure that there is sufficient room between each piece of equipment for children to run. If there are trees in the playground area, be sure that roots aren't protruding over which a child could trip. Sandboxes are a particular concern as animals can enter at night and leave feces. Check the cleanliness of the sandbox carefully.

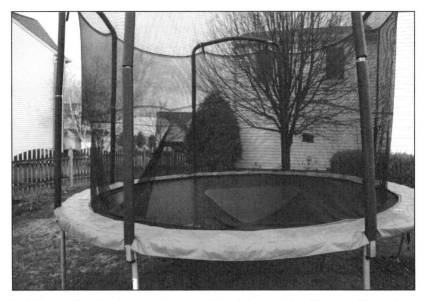

This trampoline has become torn over the winter months. No one will use it until it's fixed; however, I don't recommend having trampolines at all, since they are so unsafe.

It's easy to become distracted from watching your child—for example, while talking to another parent, texting, or reading a book—but it's critical you keep your full attention on your child at all times. While you should have your phone with you in case of an emergency, keep it in your diaper bag or purse to avoid the temptation of texting or making calls. As kids get older, they want to try more dangerous things. Be sure that they are playing on equipment that matches their abilities.

This is definitely a place where you want to have your first aid items at the ready. Keep a "playground kit" that you can pop in your diaper bag that includes Band-Aids, wipes to clean away dirt, first-aid spray such as Neosporin NEO TO GO, an ice pack, an antihistamine such as Children's Benadryl in case of a bee sting, and plenty of tissues. Make sure that you're familiar with the community and know the quickest way to the local hospital in case of a true emergency.

Pools and Beaches

I am, without a doubt, a summer girl. I love the warmth and sunlight, and I love the ocean! For me, there's nothing better than spending a day at the beach reading a book and relaxing. Of course, once you have kids, a day at the beach isn't always, well…a day at the beach. There is no such thing as relaxing. Whether it's building a sand castle, burying a sibling (and hoping they leave her head sticking out), or heading off to find a bathroom, typical children's activities at the beach turn the day into something of a marathon. The key to enjoyment is accepting the fact that, just like a vacation with kids, it's not about you, it's about them.

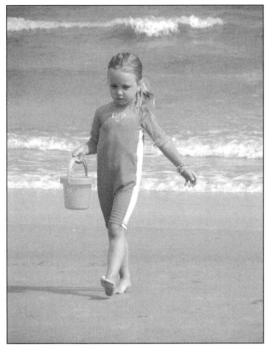

Kids are serious about their summer fun.

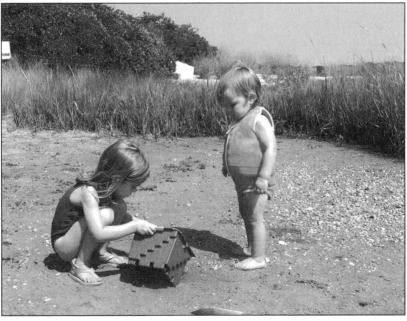

Drowning Prevention

Beaches, lakes, pools, and other swimming areas are fraught with the danger of drowning. Drowning is the second leading cause of unintentional-related injury deaths for children ages 1 to 14. More than one in five fatal drownings occurs with children under the age of 14, and for every child who dies, another four are treated in emergency rooms for serious injury. Near-fatal drownings can lead to brain injuries that can cause permanent damage. Nearly all children who require cardiopulmonary resuscitation (CPR) die or are left with severe brain injury. It's important to point out that there has been tremendous progress in the use of umbilical cord blood stem cells in the treatment of brain damage from drowning, which is yet another compelling reason to consider storing your child's cord blood.

Sadly, proper supervision at beaches and pools is one area in particular where parents and caregivers become complacent. There are a variety of reasons for this, including being distracted by another child, becoming engaged in a conversation with another adult, falling asleep, texting, talking on the phone, and checking emails, as well as the misguided belief that if a lifeguard is on duty, they're protected. The truth is that you can't always rely on a lifeguard. It's estimated that more than 100 drownings occur every year when a lifeguard is present. While many lifeguards do a wonderful job and are trained properly, distractions do occur—for example, they may be putting pool equipment away or changing shifts. It's up to a parent or caregiver to be constantly alert.

I've personally witnessed too many times when parents are totally ignoring their child as they read their book or talk on the phone. Of all preschoolers who drown, 70 percent are in the care of one or both parents at the time of the drowning, and 75 percent are missing from sight for five minutes or less.

For many years, there has been an ongoing, heated debate regarding whether giving a toddler swim lessons is beneficial or harmful. Some believe that swim lessons at a young age make the child overly confident and decrease their fear of water, while at the same time making parents more complacent. Others feel that "throwing their babies" in at an early age will help them learn to swim sooner. In 2009, a study was completed by the Eunice Kennedy Shriver National Institute of Child Health and Human Development that examined the relationship between swim lessons and drowning. It found that those who could float on their backs for more than 10 seconds and had taken swim lessons were less likely to drown.

Many parents will put swimming aids, such as water wings or floaties, on their kids and feel that they are safe. Swimming aids are not replacements for life vests! Pediatricians, lifeguards, and other safety professionals will tell you that water wings are not only dangerous, but give a false sense of security. Water wings and other swimming aids can deflate, your child could slip out, and if your child jumps in the water and goes under, they could come off. Children could forget they don't have the swimming aid on and jump in the water. The function of inflatable swim aids is to help your child learn to swim, not to prevent drowning.

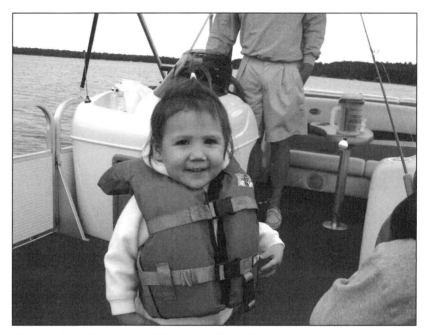

Always, always have your children in a life vest!

It's vital that parents remain vigilant and alert at all times around a pool. If you need to take one child to the bathroom, have the other one come along as well. When you're at a pool or beach and it's crowded, station yourself right near the edge so your view of your child in the water won't be obstructed. If you are at a pool party, it's easy to assume that your partner is watching your child and have your partner think you are. Distractions occur too easily. Give yourself a visual reminder, such as a bracelet or necklace that the person who is in charge of watching the kids wears. Most importantly, if you've gotten to this point in your life and you don't know how to swim, please take a lesson. You need to be able to assist your child in the event of an emergency.

DID YOU KNOW? DID YOU KNOW? DID YOU KNOW?

Staying Alert Can Save a Life

The majority of children who survive (92 percent) are discovered within two minutes following submersion, and most children who die (86 percent) are found after 10 minutes.

DID YOU KNOW? DID YOU KNOW? DID YOU KNOW?

Pool Drains

It's up to a parent to check that local swimming pools are adhering to safety rules and guidelines. Of particular concern are the drains in pools. In 2002, a seven-year-old girl, Virginia Graeme Baker, drowned after she was trapped underwater by the powerful suction from a hot tub drain. Two men pulled so hard to try to free her that it actually broke the drain cover. While the official cause of death was listed as drowning, it was really caused by entrapment due to a faulty drain cover.

Her death led to the enactment of the Virginia Graeme Baker Pool & Spa Safety Act, signed into law in December 2007. This law now requires public pools and spas to have safety standards in place regarding their drains and barriers around the pool to prevent a child from gaining access without an adult's knowledge. Safe drains have a dome or pyramidal shape to them. Drains that are flat are the ones that pose the danger so be sure to look at any pool or spa drain prior to allowing your child to go in.

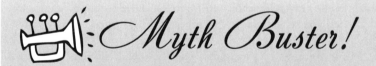

Eating and Drowning

Myth: You must wait 30 minutes after eating to swim.

This myth was based on the notion that blood will be diverted to your digestive tract and away from your arms and legs when you need them for swimming. According to experts at Duke Health, while it's true that the body does supply extra blood, it's not enough to prevent your other muscles from functioning properly. Yes, you might get mild cramping but nothing else. It's perfectly safe to go swimming after eating.

Surf Warnings

Beaches pose safety issues not inherent with swimming pools. Parents need to stay particularly vigilant at the beach. Kids can drift down the beach or stray too far from shore quickly. For children, or anyone who is not familiar with the power of riptides, swimming in the ocean can be hazardous. Make sure you read any posted surf warnings and have children swim only in areas where lifeguards are on duty. The most important thing to remember is that if you or your child is caught in a riptide, never try and fight against it, because you will inevitably end up being pulled farther out. Instead, swim parallel to the shore until you are out of the riptide. They are seldom very wide, so it shouldn't take long.

I've always been scared to death of jellyfish and have been known to scream at the sight of one. I've never understood people who try to catch them in buckets. While I try to restrain my reaction in front of my kids and not pass along my fear, I do make them aware that they could be stung, and it wouldn't be pleasant. If your child gets stung, rinse the affected body part with isopropyl alcohol, vinegar, or seawater, and scrape or shave the areas gently to remove any remaining stingers. Don't rub the area or rinse with fresh water or tap water. Acetaminophen, aspirin, or ibuprofen will help ease pain, and antihistamines such as Benadryl can relieve itching and swelling. If symptoms are severe, or if signs of anaphylactic reaction are present, seek medical help immediately.

It's important to be geared up for the beach. This means to wear water shoes to protect feet from hot sand and sharp objects, wide brimmed hats, and sunglasses that provide both UVA and UVB sun protection and are shatterproof and impact resistant. There are also bathing suits that have built-in UV protection.

Amusement Parks

New parents can't wait to get that photo of their toddler's first pony ride. It definitely is a keeper. Of course, by the time children are 10 years old, and you've had to visit the local amusement parks and carnivals innumerable times and spent ridiculous amounts of money trying to win an overpriced stuffed animal or plastic sword that will break even before you get home, that excitement will have worn off. Determining whether your child is ready to tackle a ride is tough. Yes, it's fun to see her on the flying dinosaur, but the enjoyment will quickly disappear if she's screaming her head off and has recurring nightmares about flying animals until she's in college. And how safe are those carnival rides?

Local carnivals make me the most nervous. Check for their operator's license and the last inspection date on each ride. Start with some easy rides—the seat on a carousel that remains stationary, a train ride, or some similar ride are all good bets. Don't force a child to go on a ride; the experience will just end in tears. As children get older, they will become more daring. Be sure that they understand the importance of riding safely and not taking unnecessary risks.

Regardless of whether it's a carnival coming through town or an established amusement park, it can be a bit chaotic and easy for a toddler to wander off. Be sure that you keep a recent photo with you, or, if possible, take a photo before you enter with your cell phone so that you have it electronically and can show the clothes the child is wearing to police or park security in the event of an emergency.

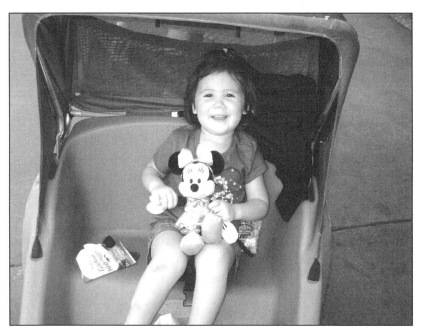

Some amusement parks will provide you with strollers or allow you to rent them, sparing you the trouble of bringing them to the park.

Play Date Do's and Don'ts

I remember my mother's puzzlement when I first told her that I was taking our son on a play date. She had no clue what this was as the word didn't exist when I was growing up. I've come to realize that not only can play dates be a source of relief, but they can also be a tremendous source of anxiety. For some mothers, play dates establish the social pecking order for their kids, even toddlers. They worry if their child hasn't gotten invited to any when they hear their friends talking about their child's ridiculously busy social calendar.

This is another area where I say…relax! While kids love socializing, they'll have plenty of time to do that throughout their life. I remember one friend telling her girls that the reason she had three kids was so that she didn't have to deal with play dates.

Play dates can be confusing at times. Each parent has her own idea of what this means and sometimes it's very different than yours. The most important thing is to have some hard and fast rules that you live by, whether your child is attending or hosting the play date, and communicate these rules to the other mom.

Parent peer pressure is a huge issue here, and you need to learn to stay firm in your rules, as this is a matter of your child's safety. If another mother doesn't necessarily agree with you or is unwilling to respect your wishes, then you need to think carefully whether a play date is a good idea. Some of the guidelines below apply to both a play date your child is attending or hosting, while others are for when she is attending.

✳ **Establish the plan.** Determine whether this is a drop-off play date and what the specific hours are. This varies depending upon your child's age and relationship with the other parent. If your child is still in diapers, chances are you'll be staying, but if this is a situation where you absolutely need to run a quick errand, the other mom might not mind you leaving for a few minutes.

On the other hand, if you are inviting a child over and you expect the other mom to stay, be sure she doesn't think this is a free babysitting opportunity and leave for several hours. Try to arrange play dates around the times of the day your child is not tired and limit the length of the play date so she doesn't get burnt out. There's nothing worse than overstaying your welcome. If your child is a preschooler, she can be dropped off for a play date (depending on her maturity level), but again, limit the length of time.

✳ **Get to know the home.** If you have never been to the family's home before, tactfully do a visual inspection when you arrive. Are there staircases without gates? Do there seem to be a lot of small items lying around that could be a choking hazard? Do you see sharp knives or other dangerous objects on the kitchen counter? If you're not comfortable with the safety of the home, stay for at least a while to see how observant the other mother is. If there are older siblings at the home, it can be distracting for the mom to try and keep an eye on an additional child. An older child's toys with small parts could be lying around, which could pose a serious choking hazard.

✳ **Find out about allergies.** If the play date is at your house, be sure to find out if the child has any allergies, so you can plan accordingly. If your child is attending the play date and she is younger than five years of age, be sure that the mom will not be serving any foods that are a potential choking hazard. While some parents know that nuts and hot dogs are dangerous, they may not consider other foods that should be avoided, including the following:

✳ Grapes, cherry tomatoes, cherries, and olives should all be cut at least in half. Grapes should also be peeled.

✳ Crispy vegetables and fruits such as celery, carrots, and apples. Carrots should be lightly steamed to make them soft and then cut into small pieces. Apples should be sliced into thin slivers and peeled.

✳ Nuts and seeds.

✳ Soft, sticky foods, such as peanut butter and white bread, can be dangerous in large gobs. (According to the American Academy of Pediatrics, peanut butter should not be given to any child under the age of three.) Spread peanut butter very lightly on crackers. Whole wheat breads and other whole grain breads carry less of a risk for choking than white bread.

✳ Large chunks of meat and cheese. These should be cut up and string cheese should be shredded.

✳ Marshmallows (including Peeps), round lollipops, Skittles, jelly beans, caramel candy, and chewy jelly candies.

✳ **Get a picture/take a picture.** If your child will be visiting a playground, park mall, amusement park, or some other public venue, provide the mother with a recent photo of your child in case he gets lost. Likewise, if you are taking another child somewhere, ask for a recent photo to keep with you.

✳ **Bring the right equipment.** If the play date includes bicycles, scooters, or some sort of riding toy, bring along your child's helmet that has been fit specifically for him. Personally install your child's car seat into the mom's car if she will be taking your child anywhere. While the mom might offer to do this herself, keep in mind that close to 80 percent of car seats are installed or used improperly. Be sure you do it yourself. Refrain from using an extra car seat that she might have because it isn't necessarily fitted for your child, nor will you know how old it is. Remember car seats do have an expiration date.

✳ **Inspect the pool or hot tub.** If the family has a pool or hot tub, be sure that it is completely surrounded on all four sides by a fence that doesn't have slats that a child can climb on. Check that there are no chairs or benches nearby that could be used to climb over the fence either. This is one of the most dangerous situations, so if you feel at all uncomfortable, stay for the play date.

✳ **Are there dogs in the home?** This is one of those sensitive areas. People consider their pets as members of the family, and it might be extremely insulting if you express concerns over their dog. But even the friendliest dog can bite if a child goes near their food or pulls their tail. The best solution might be to explain to the mom that your child is not used to being around pets, and it might be safer for the dog if he is kept somewhere else during the play date.

✳ **Plan for everything.** Bring along an extra set of clothes in case of spills or messes. If your child is a picky eater, pack some of her favorite snacks. If you are leaving, be sure to leave the mom with your cell phone number and another emergency contact in case you don't get service.

When the Play Date Is for You

Sometimes, working moms find it challenging to socialize with other moms. Most "mommy and me groups" are scheduled during the week. If there aren't many people at your office who have kids and you don't have much family support, this can be very isolating. While you might not have the time to participate every week in a play group, finding the support and "sharing war stories" helps you realize that you're not the only one with a baby who won't sleep in her crib or wondering how to get your child to eat vegetables. Often, you need to take matters into your own hands. Look online for working mothers groups in your area and ask at your church or local community center if you could post a flyer about starting a working moms group.

Shopping Cart Injuries

We've all heard the stories: mom puts Junior in the shopping cart, turns away from him for a moment to pick up apples in the produce aisle, and turns back to find her toddler crying on the floor with the cart on top of him. This may sound unlikely, but according to the U.S. Consumer Product Safety Commission, each year, more than 20,000 children under the age of five are treated in hospital emergency rooms due to shopping cart falls. The injuries can be minor and show up as no more than a mild cut or abrasion, or they could be a more serious concussion or broken limb.

Simple measures can help prevent shopping cart injuries, or at least lessen the severity of the wound. Here are six simple steps parents can take to avoid a trip to the ER after visiting the dry goods section.

✳ Always have your child use the seatbelt or restraint system.
✳ Never leave your child unattended in the cart.

* Don't let your child ride in the cart's basket.

* Make sure that your child doesn't climb or ride on the back, sides, or front of the cart.

* Never allow an older child to push a younger sibling in the cart.

* Don't put an infant car seat in the cart's seat or basket.

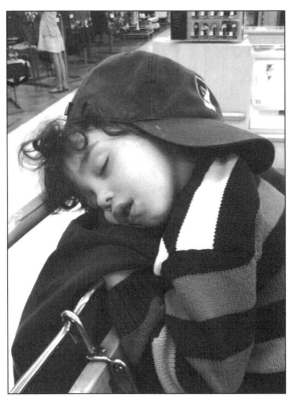

Keep your toddler safe while you shop (even when sleeping).

Organized Sports and Activities

You will quickly find that there are classes and activities for even the youngest kids. Soccer, gymnastics, ballet, and karate are just a few that accept kids as young as two years old. A big word of caution here—it's easy to get sucked into all of these activities and end up having an overscheduled toddler. Don't fall into this trap! Not only is it expensive but unnecessary. Kids need down time. It's amazing how much they can enjoy simply exploring outside and discovering different flowers, rocks, and bugs.

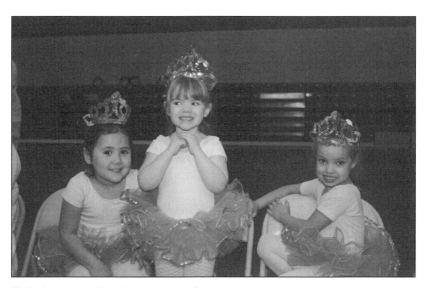

Ballerinas come in all shapes and sizes.

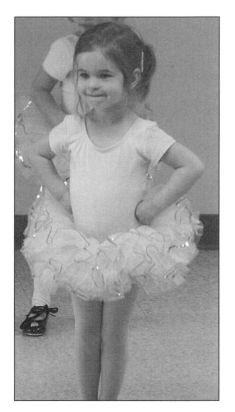

This is another area where parent peer pressure can really kick in. Just because your niece or best friend's daughter is ready for the tumbling class doesn't mean it's right for your daughter. Each child's large and small motor skills develop at different times so be mindful of her unique abilities. If you enroll your child in a soccer program, the most important thing to stress is having fun.

There are some overcompetitive dads out there who are trying to live vicariously through their children. Not every kid will turn out to be a David Beckham. And we certainly don't need another Tiger Woods, who was put on national TV by his father at age two to demonstrate his golfing skills. Don't yell at your child if she misses a goal or scores one for the other team. And, yes, if your little boy wants to take dance rather than karate, by all means let him. The most important thing is to make sure you don't push your child, and when they're playing an outdoor sport, make sure they stay hydrated.

A Word About Child Abductions

Child abductions are something we never want to think about. Some parents will tell you that they're rare and are sensationalized in the media. But the sad truth is that every 40 seconds in the United States, a child becomes missing or is abducted. Close to 80 percent of these abductions are by a family member or non-custodial parent, but that leaves a little more than 20 percent that are considered stranger abductions. In many instances, these abductors are sexual predators.

Unfortunately, while there are great benefits to the Internet and social media, it also is a window into everyone's lives. Be mindful of innocent Facebook postings that you or a caregiver put up with your baby's photo. Never include information such as last names, addresses, or other identifying information. If you're going away for a weekend or out for an evening, resist the temptation to Tweet or Facebook about your first night out leaving your child with a babysitter.

The positive aspect of the Internet is that it allows you to search a national database of registered sex offenders that live in your community. You can find it at *www.nsopw.gov*. If you're at a park or mall and notice that someone seems to be loitering, following you, or making you uncomfortable in any way, it's not worth taking a chance. Leave and report it immediately to your local law enforcement.

Taking your baby out into the world can be enjoyable, but you need to remain attentive. Public places will never be as safe as your home, so expect the unexpected.

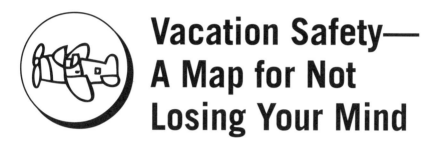

Chapter 8

Vacation Safety— A Map for Not Losing Your Mind

I don't think anyone can prepare you for how much planning it takes to get ready for a vacation with kids. There are some daring moms who will just dive right in and take their infants camping or on some other adventurous trip. For others, a family wedding or some other obligation requires travel. Whatever the reason, traveling with kids, especially airline travel, is stressful.

I'm often asked at what age it's safe to travel with infants. Pediatricians will tell you that traveling with a baby can be safe at any age, but it's advisable to avoid air travel for the first six weeks of life when babies might be more susceptible to germs circulating within the cabin. Many airlines stipulate that if you are traveling with an infant under the age of 14 days you will need to provide a medical release form. Also, check with your pediatrician prior to travel if your baby has had an ear infection within the past few weeks. You might be an experienced traveler who never has purchased trip insurance, but with kids, illnesses can pop up overnight. Trip insurance policies vary widely and can be as basic as canceled flight coverage to complete coverage for missed connections and bad weather, so make sure that you research it thoroughly.

Other than these caveats, traveling with a baby can be done at any age. But planning ahead, relaxing, and realizing there will be glitches will help make it a bit easier.

What You Need to Know Before Traveling Abroad

Traveling with kids in a familiar area is hard enough, but traveling to an international destination adds another layer of complexity and consideration. It can be great fun as well. I remember vacationing in Italy with my then 1-year-old son. I felt like a rock star we were getting so much attention! Actually, I should rephrase that—my blond, blue-eyed little man was getting the attention; I was merely the sidekick.

Proper Documentation

Be sure you have all of the proper documentation. You can check the U.S. State Department Web site at *http://travel.state.gov/visa/americans/americans_1252.html* to determine whether you need visas or vaccinations for your destination. Everyone, including infants, needs a valid U.S. passport to travel outside of the country. This now includes Mexico and Canada. Be sure you plan ahead and understand all of the requirements before wasting time standing in line at the passport office.

✳ **You must apply in person if this is the first time obtaining a passport, and both parents must be present with the baby.** If both parents cannot be present, the absent parent must sign a Statement of Consent, which can be found on the U.S. State Department's Web site at *http://travel.state.gov/passport/forms/ds3053/ds3053_846.html*. It must be notarized, and the parent must also submit a photocopy of the front and back of a valid form of ID, such as a driver's license or passport.

✳ **If you are divorced and have sole custody or your partner is deceased, you must provide proof of this.**

✳ **You must present a certified birth certificate for your child.** The names of both parents must be listed on the birth certificate. If your baby has been adopted from another country, you can also submit a consular report of birth abroad or certification of birth, a naturalization certificate, or a certificate of citizenship.

✳ **Proof of your relationship to your child is also required.** If both names are on the certified birth certificate, this will work. If not, they will require your child's foreign birth certificate with both parents' names, a report of birth abroad with both parents' names, and an adoption decree with adopting parents' names, a court order establishing custody, or a court order establishing guardianship.

✳ **A photo taken within the last six months is also required.** It's best to go to a store that specializes in passport photos to be sure it's acceptable. It must be in color, 2 x 2 inches in size, and printed on thin, photo-quality paper. It must show your baby's entire face from the bottom of the chin to the top of the head, and the hair and hairline cannot be obscured.

Plan ahead to get your passport because it can take at least six weeks or possibly longer to receive the passport. When you do receive it, print your baby's name, sign your name, and write your relationship in parentheses.

If you are traveling outside of the United States with your child and the other parent is not traveling with you, you need to have a parental consent form and medical authorization form signed by the other parent and notarized. While it's not always requested, you could be detained at the border without this document. If the other parent is deceased, or you are divorced and have sole custody, or the other parent's whereabouts are unknown, supporting documentation stating this must be provided. If someone else is traveling with your child, such as a grandparent, the form must be signed by both parents, and the medical consent form must state that the person caring for your child can seek medical assistance for your child. This form can be downloaded and printed free of charge from various Web sites, including *www.lawdepot.com*. You should also have a copy of your child's birth certificate and medical insurance card. Check with your medical insurance provider to be sure your policy applies internationally and find out if it covers emergency expenses such as medical evacuation. If it does not, consider supplemental insurance. In certain countries, if you need to be airlifted to a hospital, they require cash upfront to take you.

Packing

Packing for a trip abroad can be daunting. You don't want to be weighed down, but it's also nice to have some things from home. While you can probably find at least one Starbucks and McDonald's in the major cities, it's important to realize that the food and items your child is familiar with might not be as readily available. Trying to get a German sales clerk to understand that you want diaper rash cream isn't always easy! If you're going to be brave enough to travel internationally, you're also going to have to remain a little flexible and be willing to try a few new things. However, a few familiar foods and items will make the trip much more enjoyable for your little one.

On the same trip to Italy, we landed rather late in the evening. After checking into the hotel, I tried to get my son to sleep, but nothing worked, and he was crying inconsolably for hours. I was jet-lagged and so was he and pretty soon I felt like crying right along with him. Finally, in desperation and out of consideration for the people in the adjoining rooms, I put him into his stroller and was going to take him downstairs. Within seconds of getting strapped in, he fell asleep. It turns out that being in a familiar environment was all it took. The point of the story is that, while it might be a hassle to lug a bunch of baby gear halfway around the globe, sometimes it's worth it. If you're visiting Europe and doing a great deal of sight-seeing, be sure you have the proper stroller. Trying to take an umbrella stroller across the cobblestones of Denmark is just not smart. Invest in an all-terrain stroller that is lightweight with air-filled rubber tires, good suspension, and a strong frame. You most likely will be doing a great deal of souvenir shopping, but beware of hanging shopping bags from the handles, as this could cause it to topple over. Here are a few other stroller safety tips to keep in mind:

* Always secure the brakes when you're not pushing the stroller.

* Don't allow more than one child to ride in a stroller that is meant for only one.

* Never jog with a stroller that is not specifically classified as a jogging stroller.

* Select a stroller with a five-point harness for added safety.

* When folding up the stroller, be sure that your child's hands are not near the joints where his fingers could get pinched.

A play yard is another necessity. Safety standards for cribs are not the same internationally. A play yard will not only provide a place for your baby to sleep, but also a safe place for her to play while you are taking a shower and can't watch her.

Natural Disasters and Travel Warnings

Natural disasters might be something you've never needed to consider until your vacation. If you are traveling to a location that is prone to hurricanes, such as the Caribbean, and it's during hurricane season, check with the hotel to determine their policies on hurricane cancellations. Some will offer to re-book your stay at no additional charge if a hurricane is predicted for the days you are traveling. But obviously, read all disclaimers very carefully. When checking in, ask what their hotel evacuation plans are for a hurricane or other natural disaster. It's a good idea when traveling to these sorts of destinations to pack basic first aid supplies and extra prescription medications in case you're stranded for a few days. If you are being evacuated and you are in a foreign territory, immediately contact the local U.S. Embassy.

If your vacation destination is Mexico, it's important to realize that travel warnings have been established by the State Department. Violent crime has risen tremendously, and while a majority of it is occurring in the border towns, popular tourist areas such as Acapulco have also been affected. Use common sense when going out and stay in well-lit areas during the day. Watch out for pickpockets—men should keep their wallet in their front pocket rather than their back. Only use licensed and regulated "sitio" taxis when going out. Criminals will pose as taxi drivers and unsuspecting tourists have been raped, mugged, and kidnapped. Restaurants and hotels will call cabs for you so that you know they are legitimate.

While most food at major hotels and resorts in international destinations can be considered safe, you need to be careful in areas such as Mexico. If your baby is on formula, use only bottled water. Keep your toddler away from any raw fruits and vegetables, except for fruit that you can peel. If your child appears to have contracted an intestinal virus, it's important to contact a physician immediately because dehydration can happen quickly.

No matter where you are traveling to, leave a complete copy of your itinerary and passports with a friend or family member. Check with your cellular phone service provider to be certain you will get service abroad. If not, you can usually pay to have your service upgraded or rent a phone that works internationally.

Preparing for the Flight

Packing for a vacation with kids starts with the well-stocked diaper bag. But there's so much more. If you're staying within the United States, chances are that you can find many of the staples you use every day locally, including diapers, bath items, formula, and so on. But obviously you need to have enough to get you through the flight or drive and at least the first day of your trip. If you're flying, consider using a larger backpack rather than your regular diaper bag so you can fit more into it while on board the plane. Also, plan on bringing the following items:

* Extra diapers (plan on 8–10 per day)
* Wipes
* Non-alcoholic hand sanitizer
* Formula and baby food
* Extra changes of clothing
* Sealable bag for dirty clothes
* Extra pacifiers and bottles (be sure to have your baby suck on a pacifier or bottle of formula during take-off and landing to avoid pressure in her ears from developing)
* Extra breast shields if you're nursing
* Storage bag with ice pack to store breast milk
* A few toys to keep your baby occupied
* Laminated sheet with all emergency numbers and medical information

Formula, breast milk, medications, and baby food are exempt from the size restrictions of less than 3.4 ounces and do not have to be kept in a zip-top bag, but they do have to be declared. Airlines do request that you only bring on board what is absolutely necessary. If your baby requires a nebulizer or other medical device, keep it on board with you rather than checking it with your luggage. If your luggage is lost and you are traveling late at night on a weekend, or on a holiday, you might not be able to replace these items immediately. Also, ask your pediatrician to write you an extra prescription in case your child's medication spills or is misplaced.

Being both a business traveler and a "mom" traveler, I understand how annoying it can be standing behind a family trying to get through security with a stroller and two little ones in tow. But I also understand all too well how hard it is as a mother to navigate the entire crew through the line. The only way to deal with it is with preparation, patience, and practice.

Making It Through Airport Security

First, know that *everything* must go through the scanner. This includes strollers, car seats, and baby carriers. If your child is old enough to walk, he will need to walk through the scanner. If not, you can carry him. You will need to remove shoes, belts, jackets, and so on. If you're traveling alone, wait until the last minute to put the stroller or car seat up onto the security belt and ask a TSA official for help as the stroller goes through and when it comes out on the other end. Remember to have all formula, breast milk, and other liquids available for inspection. It's easier if you wear slip-on shoes so that you don't have to worry about buckling or tying them once you're through.

Security lines can be chaotic and crowded. Place a piece of tape on the inside of your child's shoe that has his first name and your cell phone number on it in case he wanders off, and always keep a recent photo on hand, as well as one on your camera phone. This brings up the point of "baby leashes." Prior to having kids, and even after, you might consider this horrible and even abusive. I'm often asked my thoughts on these items, and while I didn't use one for my kids, there are many kids out there who will dart off in a split second. In a crowded airport terminal, this could be nerve wracking when you're trying to make your flight or juggle all of your luggage and a stroller. As always, my feeling is that the most important thing is to be sure your child is safe, and if this gives you peace of mind and helps out, then by all means use one. I would also suggest dressing your baby in bright clothing so she is easier to spot.

After you're through security, get a few bottles of water to take on board and some healthy snacks for yourself. While they offer snacks on board, they're not as nutritious as you might want, especially if you're nursing. When you're at the gate, you'll need to get a tag for your stroller because they will take it at the entrance to the plane, and you will retrieve it when you disembark.

You Can't Make This Up

I Can See Your Underwear!

This past Christmas we were flying with my 3-year-old son to California to visit Grandma, and they had the full body scan machines at the airport. As we approached the front of the line, my husband was explaining to our son how the machine we were walking through was like an X-ray and could see what was on us. At an unusually quiet moment right before my husband went through the machine, our son announced loudly to everyone who could hear "If you see hearts on the screen don't worry, that's just my dad's underwear."

Cassie MacDowell, Connecticut

Seat, Restraints, and Regulations for the Plane

For most parents, airline regulations regarding the use of car seats and other child restraints are confusing. Adding to the confusion is the fact that most flight attendants either are not aware of the FAA regulations or would prefer to ignore them. It's important to do your homework prior to traveling and be prepared for potential disagreements with flight attendants.

I won't argue that lugging a huge car seat through airline security is annoying, but it really is the safest way for your child to travel. While most airlines will allow an infant to sit on your lap, realize that this is no different than if you were to travel in a car with an infant on your lap. If the plane hits turbulence, your child can go flying right out of your lap. The American Academy of Pediatrics recommends a mandatory requirement for use of child restraints for all children on aircrafts and urges parents to have a seat available for every child. Purchasing a seat for your infant might seem expensive, but without a doubt, it's the safest option. There is much debate about changing regulations and requiring parents to purchase seats for their infants. Experts argue that the cost would be too prohibitive for parents, and they would, instead, choose to drive rather than fly. The rate of injury and deaths from car crashes vastly outnumber those caused by airline crashes. It is a challenging debate, which needs to be weighed carefully, but what is clear is that if you choose to fly, the best way to keep your baby safe is to have her in an FAA-approved child restraint system (CRS).

An additional concern is that, in the event of an emergency landing or the loss of cabin pressure, there might not be an additional oxygen mask overhead if your child does not have her own seat. An important safety tip to keep in mind: once you are seated, count the number of rows both backward and forward to an exit. In an emergency, if the plane fills with smoke and you need to evacuate, it will be hard to see, and you will need to stay low to the ground; this way you will know how many seats to count before reaching an exit.

Airlines used to offer discounts for purchasing a seat for an infant, but many have discontinued this policy. Southwest Airlines is one of the few that still does. Certain airlines actually charge you 10 percent of an adult fare ticket for an infant to sit on your lap for international flights. It's best to book your tickets with a representative rather than online so that you understand the restrictions and fares.

Most airlines will ask for proof that your child is under the age of two if you choose to have her sit on your lap, so be prepared to bring a copy of her birth certificate. Airlines will also only allow one infant to go free on an adult's lap for one full-fare adult. This means that if you have twins and you thought somehow you could have both of them seated on your lap for free, it won't work (aside from the fact that it's extremely dangerous). Additionally, Southwest requires a Boarding Verification Document for any infant without a seat. This can be obtained the day of your flight at the ticketing counter so leave yourself additional time.

Some airlines will offer discounted seats for children under the age of two, so check with your airline prior to booking tickets.

Not every car seat is approved for use as a CRS on aircrafts, so make sure yours is FAA-approved before arriving at the airport. Your car seat will have a sticker on the side that states it is approved for use in both motor vehicles and aircrafts. Most infant and convertible seats are approved for use on aircrafts; however, backless booster seats, booster seats without an internal belt system, seat belt extensions (also known as "belly belts"), harnesses, and vests are not.

There are several vest and harness systems whose Web sites and sales material will make it appear that they are approved for flight, but once you get on board, the flight attendants will not allow you to use them. There are also some older models that might be available on eBay that have the FAA approved symbol, but these were manufactured prior to the existing restrictions. The *only* FAA approved harness device is the AmSafe Aviation CARES harness, which can be used for children over the age of one who are between 22–44 lbs. You can learn more about it at CARES (*www.kidsflysafe.com*). The harness costs about $75 and for frequent travelers, this is a great solution, but keep in mind that you will still need to travel with and check through your car seat since using a rental car company's car seat is not advisable. And remember that CARES is only approved for use on an aircraft and *never* in a car or taxi.

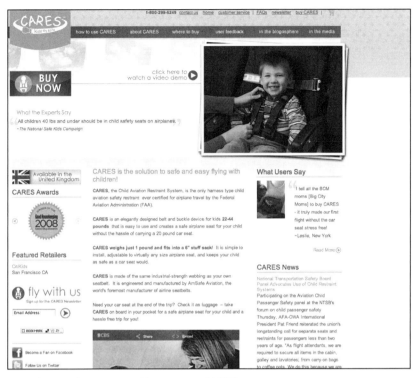

Look for a safety approved harness at CARES.

Similar to use in a car, on board the airplane your child's car seat should be placed rear-facing until she is at least one year and 20 pounds, although it's advisable and safest to keep her rear-facing even when she passes these points. Flight attendants cannot prohibit you from using an FAA-approved CRS or from placing the CRS rear-facing. It's a good idea to print out the document from the FAA's Web site to take with you on the plane that clearly outlines these rules. It can be found at *http://www.faa.gov/other_visit/aviation_industry/airline_operators/airline_safety/info/all_infos/media/2009/info09002.pdf*.

How to Secure the Seat

Securing your car seat into the airline seat isn't always easy. I learned the hard way on one of my first flights with my son that once you get the seat belt through the car seat and engaged, it can be extremely difficult to disengage it at the end of your trip. If your car seat is facing forward, twist the anchor part so it's facing the opposite direction, which will make it easier for you to grasp. Otherwise, it's flush against the car seat and extremely hard to reach.

It's important to note that a car seat must be placed by a window seat to avoid blocking a row in case of an emergency. Flight attendants will also not allow a car seat to be in an emergency row. If possible, try to book your flight for times when it's less busy, and if possible, reserve seats near the bathrooms so you'll have easier access rather than standing in the aisle waiting in line for the lavatory.

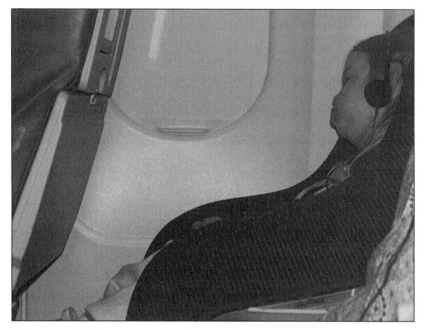

Using your child's car seat can make them feel safe and cozy in an unfamiliar environment.

Changing Diapers on a Plane

This brings up one of the most challenging issues of flying with a baby—diaper changes. Most airlines have some planes with changing tables in the bathrooms (JetBlue has one in all of them), but it can be hit or miss. So, what's the solution when you've got a stinky diaper to deal with?

Unfortunately, there's not a really good answer. Some parents use the toilet lid if there's no changing table, which is definitely an option. Others prefer to kneel down near the bulkhead where there is a bit more room. Still others opt for changing right on the seat or even the seat-back tray. Whichever you choose, *please* be considerate of the person sitting next to you if it's a badly soiled diaper. Change the diaper when your seat mate has gotten up to stretch his legs or gone to the bathroom and be sure to dispose of the soiled diaper in a zip-lock bag that you've brought along. Be sure that you have a large enough changing pad to cover the entire seat or tray and use anti-bacterial wipes to wipe down the tray. (You might also want to bring along some lightly-scented facial spray, which can mask any unpleasant odors.) There's not much room in the bathrooms and trying to maneuver with a squirming baby isn't easy. Just take the essentials with you and try to strip her down as much as possible at the seat.

Feeding Baby on a Plane

When it comes to feeding, you can get a cup of heated water to warm up formula, but warming up baby food might not be an option. It's tempting to ask for a bottle to be warmed up in the microwave, but this really can be dangerous because it can heat unevenly and cause hot spots. During landing and take-off, try to get your baby to suck on a pacifier or a bottle as this can relieve pressure on her ears.

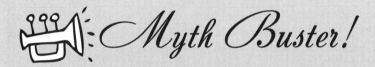

Germs and Planes

Myth: You're more likely to catch a cold when flying because of the circulated air.

An airplane cabin changes its air more often than the air in an office building. The risk of catching something due to air ventilation is only about 1 in 1,000.

Airline travel has become daunting for even the most experienced fliers. Cancellations, delays, and over-crowding lead to a great deal of tension on everyone's part. Practice some "mommy Zen" and realize that this too shall pass.

Road Trips

The famous words, "Mommy, are we there yet?" seemed like such a cliché until we took our first trip with the kids. Yes, it was cute the first time (about 10 minutes into our trip), but by the second hour I wanted to scream. I have to say, I give my parents a lot of credit. I don't know how they did road trips in my day without portable DVD players and other electronic equipment. After all, license bingo can take you just so far.

Once again, it's all in the packing, planning, and preparation. If you or your partner is one of these people who insists on pushing ahead and never stopping, you're going to be in for a rude awakening because kids have a different idea. I've always had a brilliant idea to discuss with the developers of MapQuest. They should have a button you can check when traveling with kids to calculate the real time it's going to take to arrive at your destination. I personally always add in at least another hour to my trip.

If it's a drive longer than a few hours, it's going to be impossible to keep your child from snacking in the car unless you want to double the time it takes to reach your destination. Be certain that the snacks are safe to eat (non-choking hazards), but still keep a close watch as she eats since a choking incident is completely silent. Use built-in sunshades or purchase some and be sure to apply sunscreen. Your baby could actually get a burn driving in a car for an extended amount of time on a sunny day.

When packing the car, organize everything for the most efficiency. The diaper bag and snacks should be within easy reach of you but not accessible to your child. Just as you do in your home, make sure that you have a first aid kit accessible in the case of a minor emergency.

Perhaps the greatest cause for extra hours on a road trip is potty breaks. This brings up the dilemma of potty training while on vacation. There are several schools of thought on this, but here's mine—don't do it. Sure, maybe this is the lazy person's answer, but in the best of circumstances, it's never easy. Trying to get a kid to go potty during scheduled stops on a trip is close to impossible. My older daughter was just starting to potty train when we took a trip to Disney World. There was no way I was going to worry about accidents on the plane or running to find a bathroom when we were in the middle of a 45-minute line to ride on *It's A Small World*. So, I put her back in diapers, resumed when we returned a week later, and it was fine.

On the other hand, if your child is almost completely trained and has gone for several weeks without an accident, it's understandable that you don't want to regress. If this is the case, you'll want to be sure you're prepared. Bring along several extra changes of clothing and some cleaner for the car seat if an accident does occur. Make sure that you have a potty seat accessible and that she's accustomed to using it. Introducing a new potty seat on the road is definitely *not* the way to go! Insist that she try and use the toilet after every meal and don't go longer than one and a half hours before making a pit stop.

Remember that all restrooms are not created equal. My daughter refused to go potty on any toilet that had an automatic flusher. I can't say that I blamed her—they're loud. and for a little person they seem as if they'll suck you right into the toilet. If you have a stubborn child like mine, you might have to search for a while to find an appropriate bathroom, or you can try and prevent the toilet from flushing by taking a paper towel or wipe and placing your hand over the sensor. This takes a bit of maneuvering if you're also trying to hold your child on the toilet, but it does work.

Making Grandma's House Safe

Obviously, one of the top destinations is a visit to the grandparents' house. For kids, spending time with grandparents is a great thing. They're showered with treats and usually spoiled rotten. But it's been a while since little ones have been running around, and chances are Grandma's house is not as safe as it should be. I know that even today I'm constantly told by my mother, "We didn't have all this stuff when you were a kid, and you turned out just fine."

I certainly remember jumping from one side of the back seat to the next since we weren't required to wear seat belts. While this might be the case, the reality is that, according to SAFE Kids USA, the rate of unintentional childhood injury deaths for kids under the age of 14 has decreased by 45 percent from 1987 to 2005. Unfortunately, grandparents will still insist on using the high chair or crib that you had when you were a baby. Makes me cringe every time.

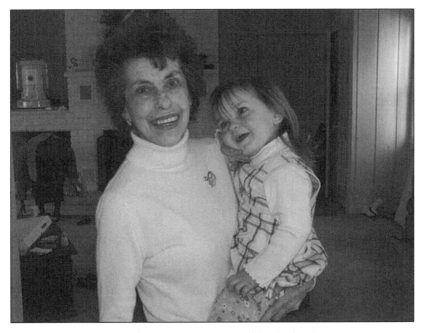

Grandparents play a vital role in their grandchildren's development.

Grandparents Babysitting

If you're going out for the evening or overnight and leaving your baby with Grandma and Grandpa, leave a detailed list of the "do's and don'ts." Grandparents might not be as aware of the importance of only placing your baby on her back to sleep. Explain to them the latest research and the decrease in the rate of SIDS since the Back To Sleep campaign. Make sure they know that they should never give aspirin to your child, even if she has a fever or cold. Aspirin has been associated with Reyes Syndrome, a serious condition that can affect every organ in a child's body, particularly the liver and brain. Many older people take a children's aspirin every day to reduce the risk of a heart attack. They might not realize that, unlike when you were young, it is no longer recommended for children.

Be sure they understand what food is permissible and what is considered a choking hazard. Grandparents are notorious for giving what they consider "treats"—items such as chunks of cheese, white bread, grapes, and caramel should be avoided until five years of age. Because they are out of practice, grandparents' response times will also be slower, and they might underestimate how quickly a toddler can crawl toward a staircase, door, fireplace, or other area.

Remind them to never leave your child unsupervised, especially since this is a relatively unfamiliar environment for your child. If they will be bathing your child, remind them to check the water temperature and never leave the child alone in the tub for a second. Whomever you're leaving your child with for the evening should be CPR and First Aid certified. If not, you should seriously reconsider. Being able to administer CPR in the event of an emergency could be the difference between life and death.

While you probably have considered and hopefully practiced an emergency evacuation plan from your own home, you need to consider what you would do while visiting Grandma or a friend's home. Even you can become disoriented waking up in a different home, and you might not quickly recall where the exits are. Keep a flashlight with you and discuss who would get the children and where you would meet. Make sure that you have the numbers for local emergency workers and a pediatrician.

Plan Ahead for the Unknown

Whether it's your mother, another relative, or a friend that you are visiting who doesn't have kids, you need to plan ahead and have some conversations to ensure that your visit is safe and not overly stressful. If you have been to the home before, you will have an idea of what child hazards to expect. If you are visiting for the first time, however, it's wise to have a conversation with the hostess prior to your arrival. They might find you overprotective, but simply explain that you want to make this trip as easy as possible and by securing a few areas from your toddler, it will make it easier on everyone.

There's nothing worse than arriving at a home that has wall-to-wall white carpets, expensive antiques, and priceless collectibles everywhere. Unless you intend to run around with a catcher's mitt and carpet shampoo, it's best to gate these areas off. This is the perfect time to use pressure-mounted retractable gates. They're easy to pack for a trip and can keep your little one out of or in a specific area. You'll also want to bring one along for the top of the second-floor stairs or the basement stairs.

If your child has allergies or certain dietary restrictions, discuss this ahead of time so that your host might be able to locate specific foods to have on hand when you arrive. Discuss severe allergies to peanuts that might require separating your child's food entirely.

Cribs and High Chairs

Sleeping arrangements should be discussed prior to arrival. If you are sleeping in a basement, make sure there is a CO detector. I once had a friend get very insulted when I asked this—you would have thought I had accused her of having cockroaches. But, as we have discussed, CO is an odorless and silent killer, which is more prevalent in a basement, near the laundry room or oil burner. If she does not have a CO detector, bring one along that you can plug in.

Even if Grandma or friends have an old crib that they say you can use, bring along your child's play yard. There's a good possibility that the old crib has been recalled, that the plastic has worn down, or that screws have come loose. Your own play yard will be familiar to them and help them sleep more comfortably. Don't forget to also pack a baby monitor if the home is larger than yours or the bedroom is at the other end of the house. If your child is old enough to use a high chair, a great one for travel is the Evenflo BabyGo High Chair. This lightweight, nylon chair folds up into a carrying case and can be taken anywhere.

It's possible that the home you're visiting only has barstools and a high countertop as its eating area. If this is the case, never attach a booster seat to the bar stool, because it is not stable enough. Rather, keep the booster seat on the ground. If your baby is young, you'll also want to bring along a baby bathtub or bathtub ring to help bathe her. Unfortunately, many of your baby's bigger items such as exersaucers are difficult to transport, especially if you're flying.

This is when a bit of ingenuity comes in. Be sure to pack two extra large blankets that can be placed on the floor and bring out some basic fun items such as Tupperware, wooden spoons, measuring cups, and so on. In some areas, you can find baby equipment rental services but always check them out with the Better Business Bureau first.

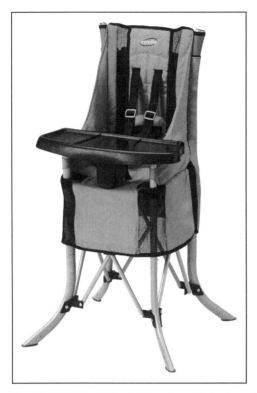

Evenflo BabyGo high chair works well for traveling.

Pets and Plugs

As discussed in Chapter 7, "Taking Baby Out—You Can't Babyproof the World," pets and babies don't necessarily mix, especially if you're dealing with a cat or dog that is not used to having their routine disturbed by the commotion of more noise and a tiny person crawling around the floor. So, it's best to keep them separated. While this might offend friends or family who consider their pet *their* baby, explain that it's for the pet's protection as well.

Be aware of "escape routes" for your baby through doggy doors or doors left ajar to allow a cat access to the litter box. Request that any pet food and water be immediately picked up off the floor or temporarily kept in an area out of reach from your toddler—another great use for a temporary pressure gate.

While I don't necessarily like outlet plugs, they're great in a temporary situation such as this. Bring enough to plug into every outlet that your child will have access to and also wire ties to secure lamp cords and other electrical items to the table legs to prevent them from being tipped over. It's also worthwhile to purchase and bring along a few sliding cabinet locks to secure some of the more dangerous cabinets in the kitchen or bathroom. Older people usually have a host of pills and medication that they will leave on kitchen and bathroom counters. Ask if these can be stored in an off-limits room and high up on a shelf. Over-the-counter medications without child resistant caps can also be nearby, so do a clean sweep of the kitchen and bathroom counters.

While some people might be proud of their incredible refrigerator magnet and wine cork collection, respectfully ask if these might be put away somewhere until after your visit. If your host has a formal dining room or table-cloth on her kitchen table, you might want to suggest pulling up the ends or using placemats instead. The old "pull the table cloth from under the plates" trick might work for magicians, but toddlers usually haven't perfected it, and it can lead to a pile of broken china and glass on the floor. There's a good chance that there might be a kitchen table or coffee table with sharp edges. You can buy some KidCo Soft Corner Protectors that can be placed on the edges and removed before you leave that won't leave any permanent residue. If anyone in the home smokes, be sure that lighters, matches, cigarettes, and cigars are locked away. It would be best if anyone near your baby refrained from smoking, due to the dangers of secondhand smoke.

Pools and Hot Tubs

It cannot be stated enough how dangerous pools and hot tubs can be. If your host has a pool, be sure it's completely enclosed by a fence. Consider purchasing stick-on alarms that can be placed on patio doors and windows to alert you if your child has walked out the door. Remind everyone that if your child is missing from sight even for a moment, the pool is the first place to check. At no time should your child be left alone near the pool. Whether they have a pool or not, it's a good idea to bring along a temporary door alarm, which can be placed under the door jamb. If the door is open, an alarm will sound.

I have a friend who had rented a beach house with her family for a vacation. Her husband had taken her two older children out for ice cream while she stayed home and napped with her toddler. A short while later she awoke to find a policeman standing in her living room with her toddler in his arms! Apparently, the toddler had wandered outside, and being in a strange environment, sat down on the curb nearby. Fortunately, a neighbor saw him and called the police.

Hotels and Resorts

Whether it's a four-star resort or a small motel, you need to be prepared to safeguard your room and the environment for your kids. Even when a hotel markets itself as "family friendly," chances are that they have not considered all of the potential hazards. This is particularly true if you're traveling abroad where safety standards might not be as stringent as in the United States.

Kid Friendly

Before selecting a hotel or resort, check it out online for visitor comments. There are some great sites that will give you information as to how family friendly a particular hotel really is. Once you're ready to book, however, place a call to the hotel rather than making your reservation online so that you can request specific accommodations. Reserve a room on the lowest floor, making it possible for easier escape in the event of a fire. It's also preferable to have a room without a balcony because there's a risk of your child climbing on furniture and toppling over the balcony. Ask the concierge or the front desk person about some kid-friendly restaurants in the area, the local pharmacy, supermarket, and even a local playground or fun spot for kids.

Inform the hotel that you are traveling with a small child and see if they have child safety kits available. If you are requesting a crib for your child, determine if it is a crib or play yard and ask for the brand and model number so you can check on the Consumer Product Safety Commission Web site to determine if it has been recalled.

Ask about the hotel's fire safety features. Each room should have a smoke alarm and sprinkler. Many hotels only have sprinklers in the common areas and some have none at all.

DID YOU KNOW? DID YOU KNOW? DID YOU KNOW?

The Reality of Fires

A small fire in an average-sized room can ignite everything in the room in less than five minutes. The combustion products from that fire will start killing people in as little as two minutes.

Check for Bedbugs

A growing concern has become bedbug infestations (makes me itchy even to think about it). You can check to see if your hotel has been reported to have bedbugs by checking the Bedbug Registry and *www.bedbugregistry.com*. Upon check-in, there are a few things you can do yourself:

✳ Carefully inspect the mattress and the seams of the mattress where bedbugs love to hide. Black spots or red spots can be feces or blood. Also look under the bed and near the headboards where they love to hide after they've fed.

✳ Never leave your suitcase on the floor because they can get in. They are not the souvenir that you want to take home! Don't put your clothes in the drawers either.

✳ Check any areas that are warm since bedbugs are attracted to heat. This could include lamps, laptops, baseboards, and so on.

Orient Your Kids

Once you've arrived and checked in, get the lay of the land. I think my kids would be happy just going to a motel down the street as long as it had an elevator and pool! I don't know what it is about kids and the buttons in an elevator, but they will fight to the death to be the one to push the "up" button. Take a few minutes to teach them about elevator safety. If, by some chance, they end up in an elevator without you, show them the button to push for the lobby and instruct them to go to the front desk and give the clerk their name. Make sure they understand that they should never try and stop elevator doors from closing by putting their hand in the door. Let them know that in the event of an emergency, they should never get in an elevator, but rather take the stairs.

After you get to your room, try to get your child to memorize the room number. Also, count how many doors there are between your room and the emergency exit. In the event of a fire, you will need to crouch down low to try and avoid the smoke, and it will be difficult to see. This will help you locate the exit. Remind your child never to leave the room without you.

Potential Hazards

Along with the elevator and pool, what kid doesn't like jumping on the beds? I can hear my mother's voice as I'm yelling at my kids to get off the beds. This may seem trivial and a spoilsport, but a concussion, sprained arm, or worse is no way to start a vacation. As soon as possible, do a quick scan of the room. Look for potential hazards, such as outlet plates, window cords, and sharp corners. Break out your travel childproofing kit to take care of these dangers. You'll also want to do the following:

✳ Check the floor for any broken glass or sharp objects.

✳ Place furniture in front of any floor lamp so that it cannot be tipped over accidentally.

✳ Tie window blind cords high up to prevent a strangulation hazard.

✳ Move all chairs or tables away from windows and ask for any furniture on a terrace to be removed.

* If your hotel room has a mini bar that does not lock, remove all liquor and foods that might be a choking hazard.

* Keep the chain lock on the door at all times. In a new environment, children can become disoriented in the middle of the night and walk out the door, having it lock behind them.

* If you are staying in a rental house or a hotel with a kitchen, be sure that there are no sharp knives within your child's reach, keep coffee makers and toasters unplugged, and remove the knobs off the cooktop.

* Store your toiletry kit, which could contain prescription medicines, hair gels, mouthwash and other toxic substances, on the top shelf of the closet. The hotel's complimentary shampoo and mouthwash should also be stored away.

* Keep coffee makers, glasses, and other breakable objects out of reach of your child.

* Take a nightlight with you if your child is used to having one on, as well as a flashlight and extra batteries in case there's a blackout in the hotel.

* If there are plastic laundry bags in the closet, move them up high and out of the way as they can pose a suffocation hazard.

* Keep slider doors that lead out to a terrace or patio locked at all times.

* Bring along a portable door alarm and window chime to alert you if your child has left the room while you are in the bathroom.

* Remind your child never to answer the door for anyone if you are in the bathroom.

When you set up your child's crib or play yard, be sure it's not near a window, cords, or a heater. Ensure that it has been set up properly and that the mesh sides are up. Regardless of whether you use the hotel's crib, always bring your own bed sheet from home. This is the only thing that should be in the crib with the baby.

Other Things to Consider

Establish an emergency escape plan with your partner. Decide upon a meeting place away from the hotel and the quickest way out of the hotel. Keep the room key on the nightstand so that you can reach it immediately. If you do need to evacuate, always take it with you. If access to an exit is blocked due to a fire, you will need to get back into your room and wait for help. When you are in a restaurant, on the hotel premises, or at any other area, always scan the room for the closest exit.

If you are staying at a hotel or resort with a pool or hot tub, carefully check the diving board, filters, and pool surround. Be sure that you never leave your child unattended and don't allow small children to sit in hot tubs because the heat can be extremely dangerous. If you and your spouse are together, agree on who is responsible for watching your child at any particular time. If you are in charge and need to step away, be sure that your partner is aware of this. Remind the kids never to run by a pool or walk too close to the edge. Apply sunscreen before going out, but reapply often if she is spending a great deal of time in the water. Similar to the points addressed in the previous chapter, if your hotel is connected to a beach, only swim where a lifeguard is present and never take your eyes off your child.

If you plan on having an adult night out and your hotel offers some sort of babysitting, either in-room or in a group setting, be sure that the care provider is licensed, bonded, and certified in both infant and toddler CPR and First Aid. Check the ratio between caretakers and children to be sure they can effectively watch your child. If your child is under one year of age and the caretaker will be putting her to sleep, make sure they know to only place her on her back to sleep with nothing in the crib but a tight-fitting sheet. Find out how they contact you in the event of an emergency. Do they have cell phones? Do they have a loudspeaker or PA system throughout the hotel?

Fitness areas are not for kids. If you want to work out while you're away, have your partner watch your child or see if there is babysitting available. As has been discussed in the previous chapter, serious injuries have occurred from children getting burns, scrapes, and strangled from treadmills.

There are some great resorts specifically geared toward families, which I personally love. Nickelodeon Suites Resorts in Orlando, Beaches Resorts in both Jamaica and Turks and Caicos, Atlantis Resort in the Bahamas (although extremely pricey), and Smuggler's Notch in Vermont are among some of them.

Whether you're traveling abroad or within the United States, you might also consider renting a condo instead of staying at a hotel or a resort. For small children, children with intellectual disabilities, or those with dietary considerations, the ability to maintain more of a normal eating and sleeping routine in this environment might help to prevent meltdowns and keep things calmer. It's also much less expensive when you can make some meals rather than eat out all the time.

Wherever you go, once you become parents, it's important to remember that the idea of vacations changes dramatically. As a mom or dad, even if you're away, you're still working because you're staying on top of the kids' safety. It's never completely restful. As I always say for parents, it's not really a vacation but just a change of scenery.

Cruises

Cruising can be a great family-friendly experience. On most of the cruise lines, there is usually babysitting and "kids camps" to keep your child entertained and give you a little time off. Before booking, check the specific cruise line for age requirements for child-care programs, as each is different. Some will offer programs for children under the age of two, but will not change diapers. Others will offer in-room babysitting for infants. Other cruise lines require parent supervision (which in my opinion defeats the purpose).

Parents worry about their children falling overboard. The larger cruise ships have plexiglass between the railings and vertical slats so children cannot get a footing. But think carefully about booking a cabin with a balcony or veranda. While most have a lock on the door high enough that a child can't reach, they could pull a chair over or climb on a table to open it. And while the railing is over four feet high, there are usually chairs and a table out there that they could climb on. I strongly recommend that if you are traveling with small children to book a cabin without a veranda.

Theme Parks

Theme parks and attractions can be a wonderful experience or a nightmare. Long lines, hot temperatures, and junk food bellyaches can make you wish you had never attempted it. Even more concerning is the fear of your child being injured or lost while you're there. Fortunately, many of the larger theme parks have tremendous safety procedures in place to ensure that your visit is both safe and fun.

With all of the distractions and noise, it's easy for you to lose sight of your child for a few seconds. Purchase a wearable ID tag for each of your kids. There are shoe tags, bracelets, and dog tags. If your child has special needs or medical conditions, there are bracelets that will list these issues as well. With toddlers, simply list your cell phone number and a secondary number with the words "please call."

You can also consider purchasing a child-tracking device or locator. These devices consist of a piece that is attached to the child's shoe, put in a backpack, or worn around their wrist. The main unit is carried by the parent. If a child wanders a certain distance away, an alarm will sound. There are a few on the market that even accommodate twins. Tell your children to find a park employee (show them the name badges to look for), but never to leave the park itself or wander into the parking lot. As with any outing, be sure to carry a recent photo of your child or take one in the morning on your camera phone so you'll have documentation of the clothes she was wearing.

When planning an all-day trip to a water park or theme park, dress for success. This means comfortable shoes that have a non-skid sole, extra socks, and some Band-Aids for any blisters that might form, a jacket in case it gets cold, and a change of clothes if your child gets wet or spills something. Apply sunscreen before entering the park and don't forget about sensitive areas, such as the nape of the neck and top of the ears. Keep a bottle of water with you, as it is easy to get dehydrated in the heat.

Many theme parks offer assistance to families with children that have physical disabilities or intellectual disabilities, sensory issues, or autism. Call prior to arriving to see what accommodations can be made. Most will provide passes for quicker access to rides or different entry points that will be quieter.

If you want to enjoy some adult rides, ask the theme park you're attending if they have a "baby swap." No, this doesn't mean you can trade in your howling child for someone else's well-behaved baby. The baby swap allows one parent to ride a ride while the other parent stands to the side of the entrance and holds the baby. When the ride is over, the other parent will be able to ride without having to wait in line again.

Beware of some rides that will appear to be easy and fun for little ones, but will actually have them screaming in terror for hours. This is especially true of tunnel rides where you really can't see from the outside what is involved. Perhaps take a "test ride" alone first to check it out.

While most theme parks try to offer some healthy and nutritious options, good snacks for the kids can be hard to come by. Be sure to bring along some healthy snacks and fruit for your kids or you risk a sugar meltdown halfway through the day.

There are tons of great theme parks to choose from, but, of course, the Holy Grail is Disney. I don't know what's more fun, experiencing Disney as a kid or seeing it through the eyes of your child. It truly is magical and an experience you'll never forget. The biggest mistake parents make when "doing Disney," or another theme park for that matter, is trying to cram too many activities into the vacation. There's nothing worse than spending a ton of money and ending up with a cranky child who's overwhelmed.

Building breaks into your day will make it easier on everyone. Disney really understands this and created Baby Care Centers in the four major parks where the entire family can relax, and you can care for your baby. Diapers are available for purchase, as well as baby food. They have microwaves available to warm up food as well. For older kids, there are TVs and snack areas. The Baby Care Center is also where park staff will bring lost children of any age to be reunited with their parents so it's always a good idea to introduce your kids to the area right from the beginning. It's a good idea to purchase a guide to Disney prior to your trip to plan it out. There are numerous parks, including two water parks, and it's impossible to hit it all in one trip. For little ones, the Magic Kingdom is a great place to start. This is where you can find all of the princesses, as well as the other characters. This might be the only park you get to on your trip and, if it is, just relax and enjoy it.

While Disney is a great place to visit, it's pricey and can be overwhelming for little ones. There are some terrific theme parks that are geared specifically to little ones that might be good to start with. One of my favorites is Dutch Wonderland in Lancaster, Pennsylvania. All of the rides are family friendly, and, in fact, there are several that are restricted to kids *under* a certain height. The admissions price is extremely reasonable (under $40), and it's a fun park for the "under 10" set. You can learn more about the park at *www.dutchwonderland.com*. Some other great theme parks for younger kids are Legoland in California, Sea World in Orlando and San Diego, and Sesame Place in Pennsylvania.

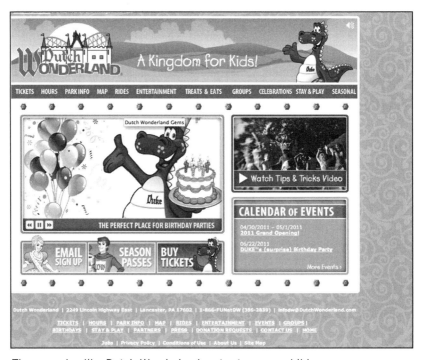

Theme parks, like Dutch Wonderland, cater to young children.

Ski Vacations

It's not always about summer fun, as family ski vacations have become increasingly popular. If you're a big skier, you're going to want to get your kids involved as soon as possible, but it's important to find a ski resort that really caters to kids. The highest priority is finding a ski resort with a good ski school. Many say they cater to kids as young as three years, but do some research online to find out about their reputations. Be sure that all of the instructors are CPR and First Aid certified and understand what they do in the event of any emergency. Do they have a PA system throughout the resort? How do they locate parents if a child has been hurt at the school?

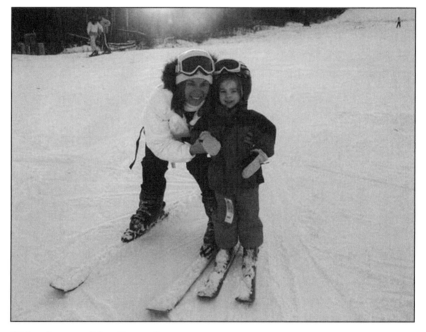

Skiing is a great family sport.

I had a horrible experience several years ago when a ski school "lost" my 8-year-old special needs son on the mountain. A woman skiing by found him on the mountain by himself in tears. I couldn't even see straight when, as I was frantically asking what they were doing to find my son, I was told to relax, it's not like it's the frozen tundra. And this was supposed to be a family-friendly mountain! Make sure that there is a low staff-to-skier ratio at the school and look for one that not only teaches them how to ski, but also helps to build confidence and have fun. Any child that's pushed too hard in the beginning will lose interest very quickly.

You also want to find a resort that offers top-notch day care for babies. Some will not take babies under a certain age or will have limited hours. There should also be a good variety of activities and events for the kids to do aside from skiing to keep them occupied. Skiing can be an expensive proposition, but it's important to invest in the proper gear for your kids, including outerwear, boots, and most importantly, a helmet. As parents, we need to set a good example and always wear a helmet. In the days before kids, you might have been a "ski warrior" and spent all day skiing and collapsed by the fire at night. Remember now that at the end of the day you'll still need to deal with your little ones, so make sure you reserve enough energy.

Taking your child on a vacation might seem equivalent to planning a takeover of a small nation, but it can be done. The most important thing is to relax, don't sweat the small stuff, and realize that even short trips can create magical moments.

Chapter **9**

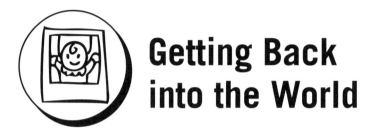

Getting Back into the World

First-time parents never realize how fast those first few months of their baby's life will fly by. Of course, the initial weeks are a blur for moms due to sheer exhaustion, but pretty quickly a routine will get in place, and in no time, you'll wonder where the time went. I've always been a workaholic, but I must admit that I got used to watching Food Network every afternoon while nursing my baby and enjoyed catching up on some reading while she napped. I also got used to not getting dressed some days until three in the afternoon and sometimes not taking a shower until the following day. At some point, however, reality sets in, and you realize that personal hygiene habits must improve, you need to wear something other than stretch pants, and the blissful cocoon that you've created must evolve. For some women, this means returning to work, while for others, it just means getting back into a routine that might include time without your baby.

I'm always amazed when I hear about parents who have never gone out, much less taken a vacation unless a grandparent was available to babysit. And for women who don't live near their family that can mean never having a date night with their partner. Not only is this not healthy for your relationship, but it will also create separation issues with your baby. Perhaps, most importantly, it's not good for *you*. The phrase "a happy mommy is a happy family" is quite true.

Taking care of an infant is overwhelming and exhausting. It's very easy to lose yourself in the process. With hormones raging and little sleep, it's easy to become depressed. And, after several months of potentially giving yourself permission to eat everything in sight, now is the time to start getting some exercise and to re-think your eating habits. Taking some time for yourself, whether that's taking a walk, grabbing coffee with a girlfriend, or a night on the town with your partner will actually help you be a better parent. Doing this, however, requires finding someone to help watch your child.

You Can't Make This Up

No, I Don't Do That for a Living!

My three-year-old has become very interested in what I do for a living. I explained to her that Mommy is a sales executive, and I spend a lot of time talking to potential clients on the phone. A few weeks later we were in a store and she was introducing me to one of her friends. She proudly introduced me to her friend's mom and said, "This is my Mommy, she's a call girl."

Pamela Speero, Malibu, CA

The Great Divide

The debate over whether to return to work after having a baby can cause some of the greatest disagreements among parents and within families themselves. Studies show that there has been a bit of a shift over the past decade to more women considering part-time work the optimal solution. Younger women are more inclined to want to return to work. How day care or outside care affects a child's development is questionable, and people can find statistics to support both sides of the argument. What is very clear, however, is that the level of quality of any caregiver situation is a primary factor.

This is one of those areas that I feel strongly is a personal decision, and there is no right or wrong answer. What troubles me is how judgmental nonworking parents can be of working parents and vice versa. Perhaps the greatest lesson I learned from my son's passing is that you never know what another person's situation is, and you can't judge. For many people, returning to work is a decision based upon economics, and it isn't a choice. There are many women (and men) who would love to be home with their kids, but need to work to make ends meet.

On any given day at playgrounds across America, you can find a host of caregivers—young moms, older moms, dads, grandparents, and nannies. The most important factor is that your child is receiving abundant quantities of love and care. Rather than criticizing another parent for the choices they are making, it would be wonderful to see everyone offering support to each other. I was so grateful to my stay-at-home mom friends when, if they were going to the grocery store in the middle of the week, they would offer to pick some things up for me if I hadn't had a chance to get food for dinner. And I know that they enjoyed my offers for an occasional girl's night out! So the only advice I will impart here is that now that you're part of the greatest club on Earth—parenthood—support the other members and realize that everyone's choices are based on their own circumstances and needs.

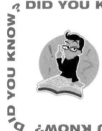

DID YOU KNOW?   DID YOU KNOW?   DID YOU KNOW?

Moms in the Workforce

According to 2009 Census Statistics, three out of four married women with children under the age of 15 work.

No, Mary Poppins Does Not Exist—Finding the Next Best Thing

My career has evolved from the birth of my first child until now. Initially, I was working full time out of a house in New York City, about 45 miles from my home. I was able to negotiate working two days from home, but I really needed to focus on working those days so it still required someone to care for my son. I was a bit naïve in the beginning and didn't really consider day care options until I was going into labor. I hadn't considered how much time it would take for me to find the appropriate child-care situation and the fact that there might actually be a wait-list at the day care I selected. After all, who wouldn't want to take *my* child immediately?

I wasn't sure whether to hire a nanny or find a day care facility. While hiring a nanny seemed like an expensive proposition, I liked the idea that there would be one person exclusively looking after my son. I had images of Mary Poppins and Alice from *The Brady Bunch* all rolled up into one perfect person who would make my life incredibly easy. Then I saw the movie *The Hand That Rocks the Cradle* and had second thoughts. I also held a secret dread that I think every other mother has—that my baby would end up bonding more to the nanny than me.

I didn't even know of any day care centers in the area and had images of these cold, sterile places that would be run more like the orphanage from *Annie* than a place that would lovingly care for my child. I was new to the area, and the few friends I had nearby were all stay-at-home moms. At this time, blogging and mommy chat boards didn't exist so I didn't have the opportunity to research any facilities online. I called some local churches to see if they had recommendations, and I called two or three neighbors who had friends who used day care. Even without the Internet, the "mommy network" already existed!

I was able to get the names of a few larger day care centers and contacted a few nanny agencies. I also learned about family day care offerings, which I had not realized existed. It turned out another option was using an *au pair*, another term I wasn't familiar with before having kids. After researching all of my options, I decided that a small family day care setting was right for me.

There really is no right or wrong answer to the child-care debate. Every family's needs and circumstances are unique. Everyone you speak with will have an opinion, which they will give you whether you want it or not, and they will be filled with horror stories about the other child-care options. The reality is there are bad situations in every case, whether you hire a nanny, an au pair, or use a day care facility. The key is to do your research, interview thoroughly, and realize that at any time you can change your mind and find another solution.

In the next few sections, I've provided some details on each option and some pros and cons. It's important that you do your due-diligence and investigate your own particular scenarios. We have provided appendices and a tear-out page to use when interviewing nannies, au pairs, and day care facilities.

Au Pairs

Au pairs are young people between 18 and 26 years of age from another country who are interested in coming to the United States for educational and cultural benefits. In exchange for being a "host family," the au pair will watch your children and perform light housekeeping duties. It's important to understand that an au pair is *not* considered an employee but rather a houseguest. For some families, an au pair is a great solution. They tend to be less expensive than a nanny and offer the opportunity to introduce your children to another culture. Au pairs are also considered to be part of the family, and many children come to look upon an au pair as an older sibling.

To really be an au pair, the young person must have an exchange visitor visa (J-1 Visa) to stay for an extended period of time in this country. There are only certain agencies that the U.S. State Department has designated to administer these visas. A great Web site to visit to find these agencies and learn more about au pairs in general is *www.aupairmom.com/resources/*. Au pair agencies work with both the host family and au pair to find a good match. They will assist with the contracts, visa paperwork, and other matters. Of course, there is a charge for these services that usually runs the host family about $5,000–$6,000. While some young people will come over to the United States on a tourist visa, which lasts for six months, and advertise themselves as an au pair in the newspaper or on Craig's List, this is dangerous for both the host family and the au pair herself.

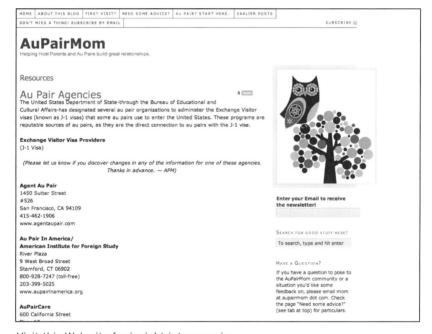

Visit this Web site for insight into au pairs.

State Department Guidelines

There are very specific guidelines set forth by the State Department as to the role of both the au pair and the responsibilities of a host family.

* Au pairs may not care for children under three months old unless there is a responsible adult present.

* Au pairs can do light housework related to the kids and cook for the kids. They cannot do heavy housework or work related to the adults.

✱ They can only work 45 hours per week, 10 hours per day. Even if they work less, you will still need to pay them for the full 45 hours.

✱ Au pairs must also be enrolled in at least six hours of post-secondary course work at an accredited school, which includes a community college. The host family needs to pay $500 annually toward tuition.

✱ Families are expected to provide the au pair with a separate bedroom, use of a vehicle, and all meals.

✱ Au pairs are also entitled to two weeks of paid vacation and at least one weekend off every month.

✱ Any au pair who will be caring for a child under the age of 22 months must have at least 200 hours of *documented experience* caring for a child of that age.

✱ If the au pair will be driving for the family, the host family must provide car insurance with a maximum deductible of $500 for the au pair.

✱ In addition to the au pair agency fees, the host family must pay the au pair a stipend of $195.75 per week.

✱ Au pairs are only allowed to stay in the country for one year, but this might be extended by several months. After that, you will need to select a new au pair.

While agencies will tell you about the up-front fees, the stipend, and the tuition, there are some hidden costs to consider. Who will pay for her cell phone and long-distance charges when calling home? While au pairs have some medical insurance, if prescriptions are not covered, you could get stuck paying these expenses. There are also just the day-to-day costs associated with having another person living with you. Don't assume that the only costs are what the agency discloses.

Challenges of an Au Pair

There are some inherent challenges in using an au pair. First, while they are not your own child, they are a young person who will be living with you for an extended period of time. You are considered a "host family" and a "host mom" and "host dad." They most likely will be visiting this country for the first time, and as any teenager or young person, the temptations are great. While they are adults, how will you feel if they are out partying on Saturday nights? Will you worry that they are too naïve to understand the dangers they could encounter? If they come from a small town and you live in a major metropolitan city, this might be the first time they are dealing with mass transit, a multitude of nightclubs and bars, and easy access to drugs. Is this something you can handle on top of having a new baby?

There are also safety issues within your home. While au pairs are required to take classes on health and safety in the home, food and nutrition, common childhood diseases, and safety and emergencies, there is nothing to say what they actually retained from these classes. Additionally, anyone who is caring for your child should be CPR and First Aid certified. While most of the authorized agencies provide "some training," they do not offer the full course for the au pair to become CPR and First Aid certified.

Cultural issues also can be a problem when it comes to safety, where safety standards might not be as stringent in foreign countries as they are in the United States. Young people might not understand the important of placing your baby on her back to sleep to reduce the risk of SIDS. She might have different opinions on foods that are safe for your child to eat. For example, would she understand that any child under the age of five should not be allowed to have popcorn or hard candy?

Language barriers can be a problem, too. While you will most likely have several opportunities to interview the potential au pair, can you really tell how well she can understand and speak English? Would she be able to get assistance promptly if an emergency arose? A good idea is to have several Skype conversations with the candidate prior to agreeing to the placement so that you have a comfort level that she can really understand what you're saying and communicate any issues.

While she might have a driver's license, be sure that she actually is an experienced driver. You might also have to assist her in getting her U.S. driver's license. You need to be comfortable that she is capable of not only driving your children around safely but also securing them in their car seats. Make it very clear that texting or talking on the phone while driving is completely prohibited. For an added level of confidence, there are products on the market now such as The Protector (*www.safetymomdirect.com*), which will prevent a driver from making or receiving texts or calls while they are driving.

Be clear as to your expectations of a daily routine. Explain that you don't expect her to be sitting on the couch watching TV or texting her friends all day long. Make sure that she understands that you expect her to remain vigilant in watching your child at all times, especially when the baby is bathing. You need to feel confident that she will remember to close baby gates at all times, not leave small toys or other choking hazards lying around, access to cords and other strangulation hazards will be prevented, burn hazards from hot liquids and flames will be avoided, and that trips to the park will be closely supervised. All of your expectations need to be clearly stated up-front.

While an au pair might say she has experience in caring for children, you need to determine what age ranges with which she has worked. The au pair agencies require additional training for caring for infants, but you need to feel comfortable that the au pair is qualified to care for your baby. She might also have different philosophies on parenting styles, and you need to be clear and up-front as to your views and be certain that she will respect and follow your instructions. For example, she might not believe in the idea of letting a child "cry it out" until she falls asleep, but if this is your plan, then she needs to follow it.

In many countries, women do not return to work as quickly as we do, and the need for pumping breast milk is not required. Make sure that she understands how to handle breast milk in regard to warming and the length of time it can remain outside of the refrigerator. You will also have to come to an understanding on the use of your car on her time off. If you are uncomfortable with her being out in the car until four in the morning, you need to be clear about this immediately.

The transitions from one au pair to another can be difficult as well. There is usually an "adjustment period" up-front where the au pair might have culture shock and be homesick, as well as having a learning curve as to her responsibilities. While many au pairs will be enthusiastic and conscientious, they know that this is a temporary position, and as it gets closer to the year ending, they can become lax. You will once again be faced with the interview process and the ramp-up time when the new au pair starts.

Sometimes, the au pair relationship just doesn't work out. As thorough as you might have been in interviewing someone, personality clashes can arise, or she just turns out to be utterly incapable of caring for your child. There are also numerous instances where the au pair has decided she doesn't want to do this and takes off, misses her boyfriend back home, and decides she wants to leave the country or realizes that Hollywood is calling her and vanishes in the middle of the night. Let's face it, they're young, and just like American kids, sometimes irresponsible. While the agency will attempt to "rematch" you with another au pair, you most likely will not receive a refund, and you will be left with a gap in your child care.

Depending upon your feelings and the nature of your child, it might be difficult to adjust to a new au pair every year, or one who leaves with no notice since your entire family could develop strong bonds with her.

So, in summary, you need to consider carefully whether you're comfortable having a young person living in your home for a year and dealing with the yearly turnover issue.

Nannies

If you and your partner travel a great deal or you have irregular hours, a nanny can be a perfect solution. Unlike an au pair, you can agree on whatever hours you require, and you have the flexibility of having the person live outside of your home. In some ways, it's easier finding a nanny because you are not required to use an agency, although many people find an agency to be much easier. You also have the ability to find someone who is more mature and might have more experience with babies. Some new parents also like having another person to provide them advice on issues with their child.

The Costs of a Nanny

Nannies, however, can be extremely expensive, running anywhere from $500 to over $1,000 per week, depending upon your individual needs and geographic location. If both you and your partner need cars to get to work, you might also need to buy a car for her and put her on your auto insurance policy. Since she is considered to be an employee, you will also be required to withhold taxes and pay Social Security benefits.

There are software programs online to assist you with this, but this can be time consuming and expensive. If you go through a nanny agency, they will require an application fee and a percentage of the nanny's first year of salary up front. Most will give you a trial period of anywhere from 30–90 days to see if the nanny works out, but after that, if she quits or you fire her, you will not get your money back, and you will be required to pay another percentage when you hire someone else.

There are online services that are more reasonable and will just charge you a monthly fee to search their site for potential nannies, but it's important to realize that, while they will do a standard background check, they are not necessarily screening their candidates but merely acting as a "matchmaking service." It's always up to you to carefully screen any potential caregiver.

While it might be cost prohibitive to use a nanny agency, finding a nanny through trusted referrals is the way to go. Stay away from sites such as Craig's List. Always do thorough background checks. The beauty of the Internet is that so much information is available for free online. A great place to start is Free Public Record Sites (*www.publicrecordsources.com*). This site lists available resources by state, including driving, criminal, civil, and financial records. Prior to starting your search, however, find out the privacy laws for your particular state. Each state's laws are different. Some require written consent from the person for whom you're conducting the background check, but others don't. If you inform the person and get their date of birth and Social Security number, you can run a check through the Federal Bureau of Investigations (*www.fbi.gov/about-us/cjis/background-checks*).

Nanny Checks

Similar to an au pair scenario, you want to be sure that the nanny has experience with infants and toddlers and is CPR and First Aid certified. Always get references and ask for detailed information about the person from her former employer, such as the following:

* ✱ What was the candidate's greatest strength in dealing with children?
* ✱ In what areas did she need improvement?

* When conflicts arose, how did she work them out?

* Was she punctual and how often did she call in sick?

* Was she good at following instructions?

* Did she ever have a car accident with children in the car?

* What was her philosophy on disciplining the children?

* What sort of activities did she engage in with the children?

* Can you describe her routine on a typical day?

The question of nanny cams comes up often. Whether it's an au pair or a nanny, I highly recommend monitoring what they are doing when you are not at home. Some people consider this spying and feel it sets up an environment of distrust. You can freely tell your nanny or au pair that you have cameras set up around the home that can be viewed remotely to not only ensure that your child is being cared for properly but also for her own protection. If there is a discrepancy with an older child, you will quickly be able to determine the reality of the situation.

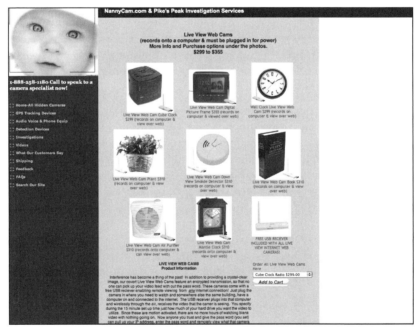

Nanny cams can be conspicuous or hidden in seemingly "normal" objects.

There are products such as the ADT Home Pulse Monitoring system, which will allow you not only to monitor your home remotely through cameras, but also to utilize motion detectors and sensors to alert you if the nanny has left the house, if she has gone into a room that is off-limits, and even whether she has put the baby down for a nap in the nursery. You can receive text and email alerts if some event has or has not occurred, such as whether she's taken the baby outside for a walk. You can learn more at *www.adtpulse.com*.

Be Clear About Your Expectations

After you have hired someone, put together a detailed list of expectations, rules, and daily routines. Even if it seems trivial, write it down. Make sure she is comfortable installing the car seat and that she places your baby in it appropriately. Explain what foods are acceptable, what time she should be fed, and that food should be cut into small pieces. Clearly outline emergency procedures in the event of a fire, blackout, or other emergency. Familiarize her with where the first aid kit, fire extinguisher, circuit breaker, flashlights, and other emergency equipment are kept. Let neighbors know that you have hired a new nanny and ask them to keep an eye open if something seems amiss. Explain to her how to use all babyproofing items and the importance of being consistent with their use.

Agree on whether she is allowed to eat your food or must bring her own. Be sure that she is in agreement with your methods of discipline and whether to allow your baby to "cry it out" during naptime or to pick her up. If you don't want your baby using a pacifier, let her know. If your nanny has children of her own or pets and you do not want them visiting your home, make this clear. Discuss what activities you expect her to engage in with your child, how much TV viewing is acceptable, and whether it is permissible for her to make phone calls or send texts to her friends or family during the day.

Make sure that you provide her authorization to seek medical assistance for your child in the event of an emergency and provide her with a copy of medical insurance and the name of your pediatrician and dentist. As she goes out in the community with your baby, she will begin forming relationships with other nannies. Before allowing her to take your child over to someone else's home, be sure that you meet the other nanny, speak with the other family, and feel confident that it is a safe environment for your child. If they have pets or a pool that is not completely enclosed by a fence, you might want to consider only allowing the other nanny and child to visit your home.

When she starts, plan on spending a few days or a week working closely with her to get her accustomed to the daily routine. Stay in the background as much as possible to observe how she interacts with your child, whether she demonstrates patience when your baby is crying, and if there are any safety mistakes that she makes.

If your nanny is from another country, her views on safety and even medical concerns could be very different from yours, and you need to be sure that not only will she comply with your instructions but will also not criticize you for your decisions. You are the parent, and even though this person might have years of experience caring for children, it is ultimately your decision.

Your relationship with your nanny is unique in that, while she is an employee, she is caring for your children and will become a close part of your family. It's important, however, to maintain a business relationship when conversations over compensation, vacation, and disputes arise. While it's nice to think that your nanny will stay with you until your kids go off to college, the reality is that you will probably go through several nannies over the course of your child's life. Don't become so attached that you overlook issues of concern and continue to employ her when it would be best to let her go.

Day Care Centers

If you have only one child, day care facilities can be much more cost effective than a nanny. Day care will allow your child to socialize with other children, establish a predictable routine for your baby (which for some children is wonderful), and provide you with a set schedule. (Unlike a nanny who can call in sick, take a vacation, or quit on a moment's notice, you know the facility's schedule.) Most day cares only close on major holidays or for severe snowstorms, but their hours are set. Most day care facilities will operate between 7:00 a.m. and 6:00 p.m., but you can find some that have expanded hours.

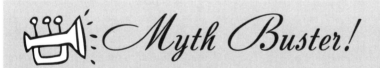

Benefits of Day Care

Myth: Children who attend day care will have problems bonding with their parents.

In a study conducted by the National Institute of Child Health and Human Development (NICHD) entitled "The Study of Early Child Care and Youth Development," researchers found that children in day care settings demonstrated a greater ability to form relationships with peers and adults than children who did not attend day care. And, in fact, children in day care exhibited more positive interaction with their mothers than did children in other settings.

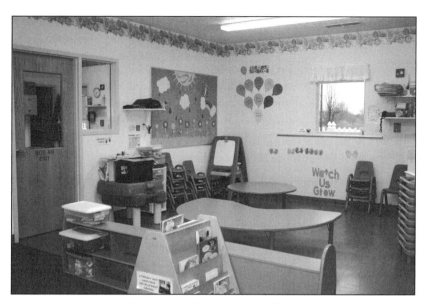

Day care schools should appeal to kids, but above all else, they should be safe.

It's important to research your options thoroughly and be sure that the day care you decide upon will provide a safe and nurturing environment for your child. Once again, do your research, tour the facility, and ask questions.

* **Determine if the facility is licensed *and* accredited.** These are standards created by national groups. Accreditation standards are most often higher than licensing regulations. Child-care programs can voluntarily become accredited; it is not mandated by state law. Therefore, accredited child-care programs have gone beyond the minimal licensing standards to assist them in providing quality care. National Association for Family Child Care (NAFCC) and National Association for the Education of Young Children (NAEYC) are two of the most important ones. The State Department of Public Health is the agency responsible for issuing and maintaining the licenses for day care facilities so you can call the Day Care Licensing Unit to check if any complaints have been filed against the facility you're considering. Make sure that criminal background checks have been conducted on everyone present in the building, including cleaning crews.

* **When you visit the facility ask to see a copy of their most recent licensing inspection report.** Make sure that all of their staff are CPR and First Aid certified and that they follow safe sleep practice and SIDS risk reduction guidelines.

✳ **Check that smoke detectors and preferably sprinklers are operational throughout the building and that fire escape procedures are prominently posted.** Fire drills should be conducted on a regular basis. What is the protocol if the building needs to be evacuated during the day—where are the children taken? What happens in the event of other emergencies such as blackouts, hurricanes, or tornadoes?

✳ **If your child is hurt, how is it determined whether he should be taken to the hospital?** At what point are you called?

✳ **What is their policy on food preparation?** Do they provide food or do you need to bring in your own? Do they have the ability to reheat food? How do they keep breast milk chilled and ensure that it is not confused with another mother's? How do they handle food allergies? Do they serve popcorn, raw carrots, or other choking items to toddlers?

✳ **How do they determine whether they will take the children outside to play?** In some areas of the country, they consider 40 degrees too cold, while other areas will take them outside as long as it's above 20 degrees.

✳ **What is their philosophy on discipline?** How do they handle a child who bites or is physical in some other manner?

✳ **Do they allow drop-ins by parents?** How do they communicate with you?

✳ **What are the classroom sizes?** How do they divide up the children and what is the staff-to-child ratio? Do they have their own cubby areas and is everything organized neatly?

✳ **How do they handle diaper changes?** Is the area clean? What is their philosophy on potty training?

✳ **Where do they nap?** Do they have a separate area with cots? Do they have cribs or play yards? If they use cribs, make sure they are not drop-side cribs that have been recalled.

✳ **What sort of toys and activities do they have for them inside?** Are they large enough that they are not a choking hazard? Are there toys that could have loose parts or small magnets? The play area should be free of sharp, hard edges, and all toys and surfaces should be clean.

✳ **What about the outside area, is it completely enclosed?** Do they have a separate area for the toddlers and bigger children? Is the surface safe?

✻ **Do they take children on walks or on trips through town?** How do they transport them?

✻ **Is the facility babyproofed?**

⁂ Electrical outlets not in use should be covered.

⁂ Any outdoor area near a body of water should be fenced and off-limits.

⁂ Staircases should be gated off.

⁂ Refrigerators, ovens, and dishwashers should be locked.

⁂ Window blind cords should be tied up and out of reach.

⁂ Heavy furniture that could potentially topple over should be bolted to the wall.

⁂ Locks should be on the toilets.

⁂ Cleaning fluids and other toxic chemicals should not be in the children's area.

⁂ Cabinets should have safety locks on them.

⁂ Windows should have gates on them or locks, which allow them to open only four inches.

⁂ Water temperature should not be higher than 115 degrees.

✻ **What type of security does the facility have?** All doors to the day care should be locked at all times. Are parents given a code to get into the building? How do they ensure that the person picking up a child has prior permission?

The facility director should be able to answer all of your questions acceptably and provide you with a list of references. Make several trips to the facility at various times of the day to observe how the staff manages naptime, lunch, and playtime. Take some time to observe the children and their interaction with the staff. Do things seem calm, and do the children appear happy and clean?

Once you select a day care, you might find that while you love the facility, the particular caregiver is not as responsive as you would like. If problems arise, keep detailed notes and immediately speak with the director to ensure a quick resolution.

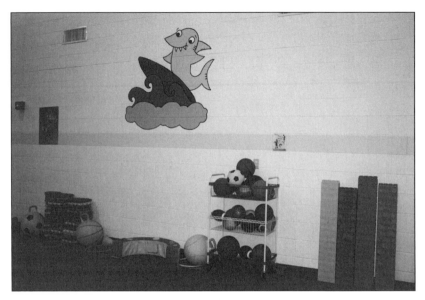

This day care facility has a gym where kids can run around and expend energy safely.

Family Day Care

I had tremendous success with family day care. Two of my children attended one and the care givers became close friends. The day care was run by a mother, grandmother, and daughter who had a degree in early childhood education. There were three other children who attended, and it was a warm and nurturing environment.

Not all family day cares are created equal, however, and you need to be sure that this works for you. Unlike a day care center, family day care providers will usually shut down for a vacation week or close more often. This can definitely be a problem for working parents. Since it is run from someone's home, there will not be as much space as a day care center. The most important concern is to be sure that they are licensed. There are many unlicensed family day care centers.

Usually these are stay-at-home moms who watch a few neighbor children. Unfortunately, many of these women don't understand that running a day care is very different than just caring for your own child. Licensing protects not only the parents, but the caregiver as well. Also, because it is someone's home, there will be more child safety hazards to consider. There might be a pool outside, cleaning products, and other dangerous chemicals in the basement or garage, windows without guards, stairs without gates, and sharp objects in the kitchen. It will be important to understand which specific areas the children have access to and how they are kept away from the off-limits rooms.

✳ **Ask about everyone else who lives in the home or visits because you need to be sure that they all have had background checks.** Find out when they had their last inspection by the state and ask for a copy of the report. As with the day care centers, everyone should be CPR and First Aid certified. What are their emergency evacuation plans and where do they take the children in the event of any emergency?

✳ **Determine how many children they accept and what their age ranges are.** If they accept older children, find out how they separate potentially dangerous food and toys from the toddlers.

✳ **Take a look at the sleep area for the children.** Are there cribs or play yards, and are they safely positioned away from windows and blind cords? Make sure that they place nothing in the crib except a tight-fitting sheet, and that they always place the babies on their backs to sleep.

✳ **Inspect all high chairs, play yards, and other juvenile products.** Do they seem old or broken? Have any of the products been recalled, and how do they track recalled items?

✳ **Do they have scald protectors on the sinks?** Do they have CO detectors and wired smoke alarms? Where do they keep fire extinguishers and first aid kits?

✳ **Do they have signs outside the home listing it as a day care?** How visible is the home from the road? Is the outside area where the children play fenced in, and what sort of play equipment do they have? Is it free of rust, and are all screws and bolts securely fastened? Do they have alarms on all the doors and windows, so they are alerted if one of the children wanders outside?

✳ **Do they prepare food for the children, and if so, is it nutritious?** How do they keep individual formula and breast milk separated and organized?

While this is to some degree more flexible than a day care center, they still will expect you to be prompt when picking up your child. Establishing a good relationship with open lines of communication will go a long way in setting up a successful situation with your child and the care giver.

Finding a Babysitter

Perhaps you only need someone to watch your child occasionally so you can run errands, exercise, or catch a movie with your partner. Sometimes, this is easier than finding full-time care, and other times, it proves more difficult. You can check some of the online caregiving sites as they will also list babysitters, but as with any situation, ask friends or local churches and schools for referrals and refrain from using sites such as Craig's List to find a babysitter.

Always get referrals and conduct a background check. Be sure that if you are hiring someone to watch your infant, the person has experience with young children and can handle the additional responsibilities. As always, they should be CPR and First Aid certified. Be clear about your expectations. Do you only want someone who can watch your baby at home or do you want the person to take her out for a stroll or to the park? If you expect them to go somewhere with your child, how will you handle transportation issues. Is her car safe, or would you prefer her to use your car? Do you feel the person is mature enough to handle a medical emergency with your baby? Try out a new babysitter before you actually need her. Have one day where he or she comes by to spend some time with the kids while you are there, and then run out for a few quick errands.

To avoid any miscommunication, write out a list of your expectations and the rules of the house. This should include what and when the kids are allowed to eat, TV channels and programs they are not permitted to watch, how he or she should handle misbehavior, medication requirements, and bedtime routine. You also should write out whether they are allowed to have friends come over, rooms that are off-limits, food that she can and cannot eat from the refrigerator, expectations on cleaning up after meals, rules on talking on the phone, and so on. Needless to say if your child is an infant, the instructions should be even more detailed, including stressing only to place the baby on her back to sleep in the crib and not putting any blankets, pillows, or stuffed animals in the crib.

Also, be clear on payment. This differs greatly depending on the number of children being watched and the area of the country, but be clear whether you are paying babysitters for their drive time or giving them gas money.

Review your emergency evacuation plans with them. Where should they go if there is a fire? Is there a neighbor they should contact and do they have that number in case of emergencies? Point out where the fire extinguishers, first aid kit, and flashlights are kept. If you have a security system, be sure they know what to do if they trip it by coming in the door accidentally, and that they know how to set it if they're going out with the kids to the park or somewhere else.

Sometimes, you luck out, and you find the perfect situation and person immediately. Unfortunately, this is rarely the case. The key is to remain flexible, be willing to explore all options, and remain focused on finding the perfect solution for you and your family.

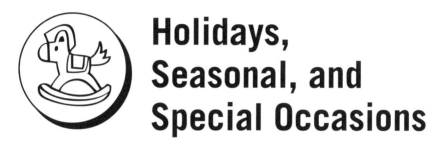

Chapter 10

Holidays, Seasonal, and Special Occasions

There are those times in your child's life that you want to make everything about that particular day as special as possible. Holidays, birthdays, and simple things like the first snowfall and the first day at the beach are just a few of them. Each of these can be filled with incredible memories, but they also can end up being the story that's told for years later of how little Johnny ended up in the hospital. Keeping some safety tips in mind while you're creating those picture-perfect moments will go a long way toward making sure everyone remembers them fondly.

Christmas and Hanukkah

Christmas takes on an entirely different meaning once you have kids. Suddenly, you become this lunatic trying to create the Norman Rockwell version of the holiday. The incessant, urgent countdown from the media, reminding you that you only have 5 MORE DAYS to get everything done certainly doesn't help. I've put so much pressure on myself in previous years attempting to create a Christmas day that only Martha Stewart could pull off that I've wound up curled up in a heap on Christmas day, nursing an eggnog under the impeccably designed Christmas tree.

I think we all have to get one of these unrealistic Christmas holidays under our belt before we sit back and realize that we're putting undue pressure on ourselves. Sure, we want to send out the perfect holiday card, make four dozen cookies from scratch, and color coordinate all of our wrapping paper, but by St. Patrick's Day, not one of our friends or family members will recall all of this effort.

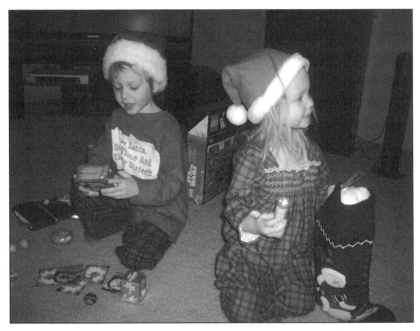

It's the feeling that is created and the simple things that count for kids.

You Can't Make This Up

"Mommy, Is Santa drunk?"

One year, a few days before Christmas, my husband and I were driving home from a party with our three-year-old in the back seat. We were shocked when we looked out the window to see a guy dressed as Santa Claus swaying down the sidewalk with a liquor bottle in his hand. I tried to distract my daughter, but she saw him and wondered why Santa was walking down the street. I explained to her that he was probably out "getting some fresh air." My husband laughed and under his breath commented that "Santa's going to have one heck of a hangover tomorrow morning." On Christmas Eve, before my daughter went to bed, my mom was helping her put out cookies and milk for Santa and carrots for the reindeer when my daughter turned around and said "Grandma, I don't think milk is going to cut it this year. What can we leave to help Santa get over his hangover?"

Stacey Kannenberg, Fredonia, WI

The "new" traditions that seem to pop up every year are what really kill me. My seven-year-old breathlessly came home from school this year and told me about the elf that comes to visit every night. No, not the ridiculous Elf on the Shelf that ended up in all the stores this year (although that one made me nuts as well). No, this elf was much more devious. My daughter had gotten it on good authority (her best friend) that if you put out a shoe near your bedroom every night in December and put a note in it regarding a present you would like, an elf would bring it to you. Apparently, her best friend put out a note asking for diamond earrings, and a pair appeared in her sneaker that very next day. I kid you not. So now, along with the presents from Santa and mom, I had to assist some 6" little man in green tights that was supposedly going to be bringing presents. Where do they come up with this stuff?!

At some point, parents will reach Christmas overload, but in the process, you can end up making yourself, your partner, and even your kids miserable. Bridezilla has nothing on a mom who is trying to fight the crowds to just get that *one* gift that every four-year-old must have. If I've learned nothing else in my parenting years, it's that we as moms always think we need to do more than we have to in order to keep our kids happy. Here's a news flash—your kids will be just as happy with Pillsbury Christmas tree cookies that they can cut and put in the oven as they would with chocolate chip cookies made from scratch that will take you twice as long!

We remember nostalgically the Christmases from our own childhood and want to continue certain traditions, but what we're really remembering is the *feeling* we had—the enjoyment of being together and the wonder of seeing presents under the tree. Yes, it's wonderful to preserve holiday traditions from our parents, but I've worked very hard to create new traditions that the kids enjoy and fit into my lifestyle. Does this make me a slacker mom? Possibly. But I've learned that by taking some things off my plate and being less stressed, my kids and I end up having a much more enjoyable time.

The other problem of adding this additional work into an already crammed schedule is that you end up cutting corners and making mistakes. How many times have you been in a mall on Black Friday and seen parents so preoccupied that they don't even notice their child wandering away? Safety concerns are even greater during the holiday season. Additional items around the house, crowded malls, and more people visiting provide dangerous situations that don't normally exist. Take a second to breathe, focus, and possibly modify some of the original plans you had.

Christmas Trees

Once you have kids, it's a good idea to do away with expensive, breakable ornaments for several years. Little ones can create homemade ornaments and paper garlands that will make tree trimming even more special. Keep ornaments off the lower branches that children can grab and put in their mouths. Never string more than three sets of lights together and a maximum of 50 bulbs for screw-in bulbs on a single extension cord because this could overload the outlet and result in a fire. Read manufacturer's instructions for the number of LED strands to connect. You can purchase a special tree cord that runs up the base of the tree and has outlets along the way so that each string can be plugged in individually. Replace any string of lights with worn or broken cords or loose bulb connections.

Secure the tree to a wall by screwing eye-hooks into the wall, looping green twine around the center of the tree, and tying it to the hooks. While I love the smell of a fresh Christmas tree, for many reasons, I have switched to an artificial one. First, trees are ridiculously expensive, and I personally have a hard time thinking about all of the trees that are cut down every year. Secondly, they are a pain to clean up every year and having stray pine needles lying around with a toddler isn't fun.

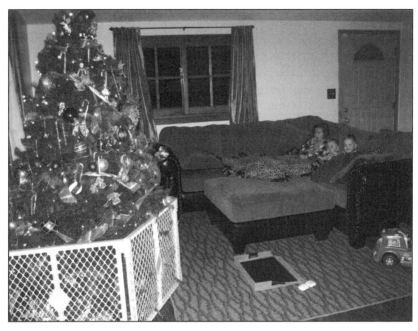

If you can't secure the tree, you can always gate it off.

DID YOU KNOW? DID YOU KNOW? DID YOU KNOW?

Christmas Tree Fires

Every year fire departments respond to approximately 260 fires caused by Christmas trees. One of every 21 reported fires that began with a Christmas tree resulted in death.

Never leave a tree lit when leaving the house or going to bed and be sure there is always water in the base. Be sure that the tree is not near a heat source because this is one of the primary causes for Christmas tree fires. I've now purchased "Christmas tree" spray, and my artificial tree looks so realistic most people don't realize it's not a live tree.

Menorahs

Make sure that you place the menorah out of reach of kids and pets. Excited children could accidently knock it down and if they go to blow out the candles, hot wax could splatter on them. Also, consider the placement of it. If you will be placing it in a window, make sure that curtains and drapes are pulled back. Be sure that the window you select does not have a couch underneath it where it could ignite the fabric if the menorah fell onto it.

Decorations

Some of the decorations that have been passed down to you from your family might be becoming old and frayed. Check for loose parts or frayed electrical wires. Glass and ceramic items should be placed high up out of reach of kids. Never use candles for decorations! There are now battery-operated flameless candles that are just as beautiful and much safer. Any decorations that plug into a wall are dangerous. The cords need to either be attached to the wall or secured to the side of a table leg.

Small pieces from Christmas villages or nativity scenes can definitely be a choking hazard—you don't want your baby trying to eat one of the Wise Men. Shiny objects and lit decorations can capture your child's attention. Even if you place these items high up on shelves or cabinets, a child can easily pull a chair or bench over to try and stand and reach them, potentially causing everything to topple over on him. Avoid any objects that might cause temptation for your child.

Party Patrol

More than likely, you will be entertaining during the holidays and people, especially older relatives, who are not familiar with the numerous dangers toddlers can get into, might not be prepared. Secure a room or closet to keep guests' purses and bags that can be off-limits to your child. Medications, matches, and candy that might be in someone's purse can be dangerous if your child accidently goes through it. If a guest presents your child with a gift, check that it is an age appropriate item that doesn't present any choking or strangulation hazards.

Whether you are hosting a party or attending one, make sure that any food that is laid out is safe for your child. Items such as nuts, party platters of cubed meats and cheeses, and raw carrots are all potential choking hazards. While you can't ask a hostess to remove all of her food, do not let your child out of your sight. Choking can happen in a matter of seconds and is silent. If several people are talking and music is playing, you could be completely oblivious that your child is choking. This might be another instance where you and your partner take turns being in charge of watching your child.

Be alert for half-filled glasses of alcoholic beverages left unattended on a table as well. Most importantly, if you are attending a party, decide on a designated driver. Don't drink and drive! If you're having an elegant dinner party, consider using festive place mats rather than a tablecloth because your child can try the old magic trick of pulling it right off the table. (No, the fine china and crystal will not remain on the table!) Again, flameless candles are the safest way to go.

Holiday Baking

I will admit I'm not "Suzy Homemaker." While I love to cook, I fall short in the baking category and can barely manage a tray of brownies. If you, however, are one of those "Domestic Goddesses" I read about and love nothing more than baking dozens of tins of Christmas cookies, your kids will love getting involved. The key is to find age-appropriate tasks for them and maintain a watchful eye.

Some great jobs for kids include rolling out the dough, using cookie cutters to make the shapes, and decorating them once they're out of the oven. Make sure you set up a workstation in a safe area away from the stove, electrical appliances, and sharp knives. Constantly remind your child about the importance of good hand washing and to clean up work areas. Never leave kids unattended around the oven and be sure that everyone is aware of the location of fire extinguishers in the house.

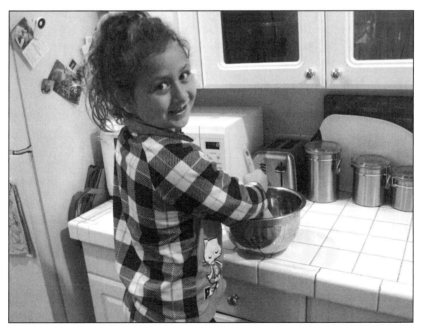

Helping out with the baking makes it festive for everyone.

Toys

It's hard to say *no* to your little angels when they're begging for the latest, greatest, must-have, absolutely will-die-without toy that is advertised 24/7 during the holiday season. I've decided there's a special place in hell reserved for advertising and public relations (PR) execs execs that hype these items to kids. We can make ourselves crazy almost going to battle with another mother over the last available Dancing Dora doll. The reality is that sometimes that "must-have" toy is really not appropriate for our kids. Every year we see a list of the most dangerous toys of the season, but there are many more that, while they might be appropriate for another child, are not age appropriate for yours. This is where you sometimes have to make those tough decisions as a parent and do what's safe rather than what's popular.

Several years ago we saw thousands of toys recalled around the holiday season due to lead paint and other issues. Parents became frustrated and confused as to what was and was not safe to buy. While major retailers were quick to pull recalled products off the shelves, many unsafe items remained in discount stores and online. It seemed as if another toy was being recalled every day, and if you had already bought one of those toys, all of a sudden you were out of luck if it was recalled the next day. Most importantly, read the age requirements of any toy and believe them! Yes, you might feel that your 3-year-old really does have the maturity to play with a toy that's labeled for a 6-year-old and above, but there's a reason that label is on there.

When your child receives a toy as a gift, check the Consumer Products Commission Web site to be sure that it hasn't been recalled. If there is a manufacturer's warranty card, immediately fill it in and send it back so you will be alerted to any recalls. Carefully inspect the toy to be sure there are no choking and strangulation hazards present. Great Aunt Edna might not understand which toys are or are not appropriate for a young child.

Button battery ingestion is a growing problem and increases around the holidays as parents are installing batteries into new toys and games. Batteries can get stuck in a child's throat and esophagus and could create an electrical current or chemical burn. A burn can happen even if the battery is not "leaking" or damaged and can occur within two hours of ingestion.

Along with toys, consider other products with small batteries, such as cameras and singing greeting cards. Avoid toys with magnets and small parts for smaller children. Both of these present serious choking hazards for children. Additionally, magnets, if ingested, can cause perforations to the intestine or can become attached, causing blockage, holes, or even poisoning. This isn't just a danger for small children, however, as boys as old as 11 years of age have been treated for magnet ingestion, according to the Consumer Products Safety Commission. If your child gets any sort of riding toy, make sure that you provide a helmet to go along with it.

Shopping Safety

Shopping during the holidays alone is stressful enough, but with a toddler or two in tow, it can be enough to put you over the edge. The key is to remain realistic and keep the excursion limited to a reasonable amount of time. Over-tired and over-hungry kids will leave you stressed out and tense. It's not worth trying to push it and fit in just one more errand. Consider shopping with a friend who can help keep an eye on your kids in case you want to try something on or while you're standing in the checkout line. This could also allow you to drop the kids off with a friend at the front of the mall so they can leave their coats in the car. An over-heated kid is no better than an over-tired or over-hungry one. Make sure before you even enter the mall you review basic safety facts with your kids:

✱ Remind them that you expect them to stay with you at all times and not wander off. If they see something interesting, they should tell you they want to stop and look at it.

✱ Be sure they know their home phone number and your cell phone number and tell them that if they get lost to find a "mommy" to ask for help.

✱ Remind them never to leave the store if they get lost in it, because you won't leave either until you find them.

Trying to get a baby out of a car and secured into a stroller while your toddler is trying to crawl out makes you wish you really did have those proverbial eyes in the back of your head. A good trick is to teach your older kids to keep one hand on the car as you're getting the baby settled in the stroller. Never allow your child to run ahead of you in a parking lot because someone backing out might not see him.

While the ordeal of trying to get kids out of the car and strapped into a stroller is certainly daunting, resist the urge to leave them in the car, even for just a few minutes while you run in for a quick errand. Every year, hundreds of kids are involved in potentially fatal accidents being left in cars. Children have been able to shift the car into gear, gotten limbs and even their necks caught playing with windows, and suffered hypothermia. In some states, it can be considered a misdemeanor offense to leave a child alone in a car and can be upgraded to a felony if an injury occurs. Most parents never imagine that a tragedy will occur and assume if they're just running in to pick up dry cleaning or return a library book, their children will be fine, but these accidents can occur in a matter of minutes. Either delay your errand until you're alone, or take your kids with you.

In the mall many distractions, such as carolers and, of course, Santa Claus, are on hand to entice a child to stray away from their parents. This brings up another point. While every parent can't wait for that first photo of their child sitting on Santa's lap, don't force the issue. You'll only end up with paying for an over-priced photo of a screaming child.

What to Do When Your Child Gets Lost at the Mall

If your child does get lost, immediately report it to the nearest store clerk and security guard. Don't be embarrassed to yell loudly that your child is missing. Any embarrassment on your part is minor compared to the regret you'll feel if something has happened to your child. While most children are lost for only a few minutes, sadly child abductions happen every day, and the added crowds and confusion at stores during the holidays makes it that much easier.

Many stores now participate in "Code Adam." This is a program that was originally created by Walmart to help locate missing children who are either lost or have been potentially kidnapped from a retail store. It's named after Adam Walsh, the 6-year-old son of John Walsh, host of *America's Most Wanted* TV show. Adam was abducted from a Sears in Florida in 1981 and later found murdered.

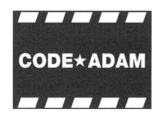

Look for this Code Adam symbol at stores.

Today, many retail stores, movie theaters, amusement parks, and other buildings utilize Code Adam, and in 2003, Congress mandated that Code Adam be implemented in every federal office building. If a store participates in Code Adam, they will have this information posted on the door or near the courtesy desk. Essentially, Code Adam works like this:

✻ If your child is missing, locate a store employee and tell him that you want the store's assistance in finding your child. Provide them with as much detail about your child as possible, including his name, age, ethnicity, height, weight, eye color, hair color, and what he was wearing.

✻ The employee will immediately have a Code Adam announced over the public address system with the description of your child. They will *not* mention his name because that could help a potential abductor even further to lure your child out of the building.

* While Code Adam protocol does not stipulate that the store is immediately locked down, some have been known to do this. Usually, the greeter at the front of the store monitors everyone entering and exiting the building, and if it's a big box store, an employee is stationed at every exit. All other employees within the store will immediately start searching inside as well as the parking lot.

* If the child is not located within 10 minutes, the local police are called.

* If the child is found accompanied by someone other than the parent or guardian, employees will make a reasonable effort to delay their departure, provided it does not put the employee(s) or child at risk. They will definitely get as much detailed information as possible, including a description of the person and make, model, and license plate of the car.

* If the child is found simply lost and unharmed, they are reunited with the adult searching for them.

* The Code Adam is cancelled over the same storewide communication system used to initiate it, either because the child has been reunited with the searching adult or the police have arrived and taken over the situation.

Escalators

Getting lost isn't the only hazard at malls. Escalators can be extremely dangerous as well. Every year there are nearly 1,000 escalator injuries. The majority of these happen to children under the age of six. Injuries can include mangled hands and feet, lacerated tendons, broken or cut-off fingers and toes, and head injuries. In some cases, escalator injuries occur when children get their hands caught between moving and stationary parts of the handrail or shoe laces caught between the steps. Others are hurt while playing at the foot of the escalator and becoming entangled in the machinery of the comb plate at the bottom of the stairs.

Before getting onto an escalator, check for loose or dangling items of clothing. Shoelaces, mittens, and drawstrings can get trapped in an escalator's moving parts. Lift toddlers on and off the step. Shoes and boots with soft rubber soles have been known to slip into cracks between steps and the escalator wall, so try to keep those little feet planted firmly on the step. Never take a stroller onto an escalator. Again, you might be impatient waiting for a crowded elevator, but don't take the risk. Escalator steps aren't wide enough to accommodate a stroller, so its weight may not be evenly balanced on the step; if the stroller tips over, you and your baby could take a nasty tumble. If your child gets caught, immediately push the emergency button that is usually located at both ends of the escalator.

At multi-level malls, make sure that your kids don't stand on couches, chairs, or benches that could be close to the railing. Don't allow them to hang over the sides and keep them away from fountains.

Germs

Perhaps the greatest source of germs at a mall is in the food courts. A recent study found that there are as many germs on a food court tray as there are on a toilet seat. Make sure that you have some wipes along with you to wipe down the tray prior to putting any food on it or get the food in a bag so you don't have to use the tray.

Trying to negotiate a diaper bag, purse, stroller, and a bunch of shopping bags isn't easy. Once again, while it might be an inconvenience, make several trips to the car to drop off packages as you purchase them. Hanging shopping bags off the back of the stroller could cause it to become unstable and tip over with your baby strapped inside.

In the end, the look on your kids' faces as they're opening up presents is worth all of the time and effort, but keep it in perspective and realize that buying them the entire toy store doesn't ultimately make you a better parent in their eyes.

Winter Safety

In most parts of the country, snow is a reality of winter. I must admit that I enjoy the first snow day of the year as much as the kids. There's something about it that makes everyone feel like a kid again. That enthusiasm quickly wears off for me, though, and by the third school cancellation, I'm ready to pack it in and move to Hawaii. Unfortunately, that doesn't seem to be on my itinerary any time soon, so I've learned to find ways to make the most of it. I think the thing that makes me the craziest is spending 45 minutes getting them bundled up to go outside, only to have one of them say that they first need to go to the bathroom. Then, once we get outside, they're clamoring to get back in for hot chocolate within about 10 minutes. I've now made it a rule that if we get dressed to go outside, we're sticking with it for at least 30 minutes. I figure if I'm committed to living in the Northeast, then I'm going to get my kids into skiing and ice-skating. Getting them started young is much easier than trying to teach them once they are older. There are so many great outdoor sports to enjoy in the winter, but it's important to take some basic safety precautions, participate responsibly, and recognize when it's time to take a break.

The Right Clothes Make a Difference

The right clothes can make the difference between having fun and being miserable while participating in winter sports. Layering is the name of the game. It's best to avoid cotton because it doesn't keep kids very warm and will get cold when it retains moisture. Rather, start with a nylon-type shell and then continue with a turtleneck, fleece, and coat. Scarves should be avoided since the ends can get caught and pose a strangulation hazard. Instead, look for a gaitor (it's the top piece of a turtle neck) to protect children's necks fully.

Hats and warm gloves are a must, and be sure to keep an extra pair of gloves and socks on hand, as these are the first items to get wet and cold. Make the outer layer of clothing waterproof, because this will help keep the layers underneath dry. Sunglasses should be worn and sunscreen applied—those UV rays are still coming through!

Sports and Their Dangers

Sledding is perhaps the easiest winter sport for everyone in which to participate. But it can be dangerous.

DID YOU KNOW? DID YOU KNOW? DID YOU KNOW? DID YOU KNOW?

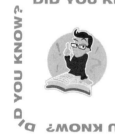

Rate of Sledding Accidents

According to the National SAFE Kids Campaign, hospital emergency rooms treat approximately 15,000 children ages 5 to 14 for sledding injuries each year.

DID YOU KNOW? DID YOU KNOW? DID YOU KNOW?

Head injuries are a common and serious type of sledding injury. Parents should always supervise their children while sledding and make sure that the hill is safe. (For example, there should be no obstacles in the path, and it shouldn't end on a pond or near a parking lot or street.) Children should wear a helmet while sledding and always go down feet first, sitting forward.

Skiing and snowboarding are great winter sports and can be enjoyed by the entire family. Children should be taught to ski and snowboard responsibly and learn the National Ski Patrol's Responsibility Code. While lessons aren't imperative, it's a good idea to start children off with one or two lessons so that they learn the basics. Both snowboarders and skiers should always wear helmets. Unfortunately, many of us grew up not wearing helmets, but we set a bad example for our kids if we don't. Only a little over 60 percent of kids currently wear ski helmets. The use of ski helmets has been shown to reduce head injuries by almost 50 percent, so insist on the use of one every time they ski. It's also important that the helmet fits properly. Refrain from using a hand-me-down or your child's bike helmet, which isn't a substitute for a ski helmet.

Also, make sure that the equipment your children are using is appropriate for their height and weight and is in good working order. Goggles or glasses should be worn and will help protect kids' eyes from sun and flying objects. Above all, set a good example for your children by being a courteous and responsible snowboarder or skier. Don't ski recklessly or stop in the middle of the mountain.

Ice-skating is another great sport that can be enjoyed by the entire family and costs very little. Again, make sure that your child's skates fit properly and provide ankle support. Do not skate on a pond or lake unless it has been designated as a safe skating area and be sure to check for cracks and holes in the ice. Never allow your child to skate alone—insist on the buddy system.

Frost Nip and Frostbite

Be sure to keep an eye out for frost nip and frostbite. Frostbite occurs in children much faster than in adults, as kids lose heat from their skin much more quickly. Make them stop and take a break frequently to come in for a warm snack and to change any wet clothes. Frost nip is less severe than frostbite and acts as an early warning sign of the onset of frostbite. It usually affects the tips of the ears, fingers, cheeks, nose, and toes. The skin can become numb and tingly. To treat it, remove wet clothing and immerse the chilled body part in warm water, between 100°–104 degrees.

Frostbite occurs when the skin and outer tissues become frozen. This condition tends to happen on extremities like the fingers, toes, ears, and nose. They may become pale, gray, and blistered. At the same time, the child might complain that her skin burns or has become numb. The skin may appear waxy or discolored, and it will be cold to the touch. The severity depends on several factors, including temperature, length of exposure, wind-chill factor, dampness, and type of clothing worn.

To care for frostbite, soak the area in warm water (no warmer than 105 degrees. Keep the area in the water until it looks red and feels warm. Do not rub the area because this can cause further damage to soft tissue. Instead, loosely bandage the area with a dry sterile dressing.

With the right clothing, proper equipment, and basic safety measures they'll be snow bunnies in no time.

Summer Safety

I've always said that I was somehow born on the wrong coast. After spending ten years in southern California, I quickly realized that I was meant to be a beach girl. I love the sun, sand, and surf. My goal is to convince my kids that they all want to go to college in California so that we can pack up one day, and I can move back.

Even just the first hints of spring make me giddy with anticipation. While I don't put much stock in Puxatawny Phil's predictions, I must admit I do get the slightest bit hopeful when that ground hog doesn't see his shadow. The greatest disappointment to me is when Mother Nature teases us in March and gives us a few gorgeous days and then ends up dumping a snowstorm on us. But when daylight savings time starts, I know we're well on our way to warmer days.

Check Equipment

My kids can sense it, too. The first day the temperature goes above 50 degrees, they're ready to hop on their bicycles and take off. Whether it's a bicycle or tricycle, since it's been sitting over the winter unused, make sure that it's still in good condition. Look for frayed cables and replace worn-out brake pads. Oil the chain and remove any dirt and be sure that the tires are inflated to the pressure that's recommended on the sidewall of the tire. Check that their bike helmet still fits them properly and, if there are any cracks or it appears worn out, replace it.

Now that the kids will be out playing when it's dusk, make sure they have light reflectors on their bicycles and post signs in the driveway warning delivery people that children are playing. Remind your children that if their ball rolls into the road, they should call an adult to help retrieve it. If at all possible, have your kids play in the backyard rather than the front where they are visible from the road. If you live in an area where a stray dog or other animal could wander into the yard, teach your kids never to approach it but to call you.

Check that swings and other playground items are rust-free and in good working order. If you store outdoor toys and bicycles in the garage, be sure that other hazardous items such as fertilizer, plant food, and paints are locked away and not accessible to your kids.

Beware of Trampolines

If you are thinking of purchasing a trampoline or already have one, consider this fact: according to the U.S. Consumer Product Safety Commission (CPSC), hospital emergency room–treated trampoline injuries almost tripled in the last decade, from an estimated 37,500 in 1991 to almost

100,000 in 1999. Nearly two-thirds of trampoline injury victims were children 6 to 14 years of age and roughly 15 percent of trampoline injuries involved young children under six years old.

Falls off the trampoline often resulted in crippling injury or death, including paralysis from a spinal cord injury. Somersaults and coming into contact with other persons on the trampoline's surface likewise resulted in many serious and crippling injuries as well as deaths. Pediatricians advise against allowing preschoolers to use trampolines at all.

Grilling and Sunscreen

Once you're ready to start cranking up the barbeque, make sure that grilling tools are out of reach and consider placing a portable gate around the grill to keep kids away from it. Food poisoning is a greater concern in the summer months when the temperatures rise. Hot weather is the perfect breeding ground for food-borne bacteria, which grows rapidly in moist air when the temperature is between 90 and 110 degrees. Be sure that foods such as raw or cooked meats, luncheon meats, and mayonnaise-based foods are stored in a cooler with several inches of ice. If the ice melts, it's important to replenish it as soon as possible.

When grilling outside or away from home, take a meat thermometer along to check that the meat is cooked completely. Especially when grilling, food can appear completely cooked on the outside but not be heated to the proper internal temperature. Keep raw meat well wrapped and be sure that if any juice drips, it's cleaned up immediately with an anti-bacterial wipe. If juices come into contact with already prepared food, don't eat the food. Whatever utensils or cutting boards are used for raw meat should immediately be wrapped up and stored away. One of the greatest causes of food-borne illnesses is improper hand washing. Be sure to pack hand sanitizer gel and anti-bacterial wipes for washing up. If you're camping or grilling away from home, bring a jug of water and some dish soap to wash off utensils and plates.

Even if the weather is just starting to get warm up, it's important to always apply sunscreen. Burns can happen at any time of the year, and the consistent use of sunscreen during childhood can substantially reduce the incidence of certain skin cancers by as much as 78 percent.

Drowning

While pool and beach safety have been discussed in previous chapters, it can't be stressed often enough how cautious you need to be with kids around water. Drowning occurs in seconds and is completely silent.

Another phenomenon that many people are not familiar with is dry drowning in which a person drowns without being in water. There is a delayed effect—between one hour and 24 hours—from the time the water reaches the person's lungs. Each year, about 4,000 Americans die from dry drowning, including 1,400 children. It usually happens with people who are swimming for the first time or those who are not good swimmers. People suffering from asthma are also more at risk. Someone will accidently swallow water or become submerged for a brief period and appear to be fine at that moment. Hours later, symptoms appear, including extreme fatigue, difficulty in breathing, and changes in behavior. All are the result of reduced oxygen flow to the brain. If your child has any of these symptoms and he has recently been swimming, you should immediately take him to the hospital.

Dehydration

Dehydration is another concern, especially for kids in the summer. Heat exhaustion or heat strokes can occur when the humidity and temperature rise and the body's cooling-down mechanism becomes too overwhelmed by the heat. When kids are running around, they might not even be aware they are becoming dehydrated. Make sure that they drink lots of water and have them take breaks in the shade. Stay away from juices with high sugar content because they can worsen the impact of dehydration on the body.

The Dangers of Lyme Disease and Bee Stings

Regardless of where you live in the country, Lyme disease has become a serious issue and is growing at an alarming rate. According to the Centers for Disease Control, by 2012 they predict there will be at least 80,000 cases every year and possibly as many as 160,000. According to the Centers for Disease Control, Lyme disease is most common among boys aged 5–19. This age group is affected at three times the average rate of all other age groups. Around 25 percent of all reported cases are children.

When identified and treated quickly, people recover completely, but unfortunately in many cases Lyme disease goes undetected for quite some time and can have long-term and debilitating effects. This is especially true with kids who might not notice a tick bite or symptoms that will appear to be a mild case of the flu. Lyme disease can affect different body systems, such as the nervous system, joints, skin, and heart. While the initial symptom is usually the common "bulls-eye" rash, in some cases, it never develops. Other symptoms could include flu-like symptoms, such as swollen lymph nodes, fatigue, headache, and muscle aches. Over time these symptoms can disappear, but there is also the potential that the infection can spread to other parts of the body.

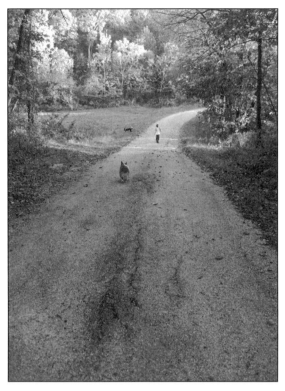

A boy, two dogs, and the woods. Doesn't get any better than that. Just be sure he doesn't bring home any ticks.

Lyme disease can affect the heart, leading to an irregular heart rhythm or chest pain. It can spread to the nervous system, causing facial paralysis (Bell's palsy), or tingling and numbness in the arms and legs. It can start to cause headaches and neck stiffness, which may be signs of meningitis. Swelling and pain in the large joints also can occur.

Other possible symptoms may include the following:

* Neurological symptoms
* Heart problems
* Skin disorders
* Eye problems
* Hepatitis
* Severe fatigue
* Weakness
* Problems with coordination

The good news is that an infected tick has to be attached to the person's skin for two days to transmit Lyme disease, so it gives parents time to remove it. They are so small, though, that it is easy to mistake the tick for a freckle or a small scab. It's crucial to check your child every day, especially at the scalp line, under armpits, and near the groin for ticks. Do a tick check the minute they walk in the door and have them change out of the clothes they are wearing. Don't forget to use tick spray or a tick collar on your pets to keep them safe as well.

If you do find a tick on your child, use sharp-pointed tweezers to grab the tick near the head, not the body, and pull out firmly without twisting. Save the tick in a jar or plastic bag until you contact your pediatrician. He or she might want you to send the tick in for testing or will tell you to mark the date on your calendar that you discovered it so that you can begin watching for symptoms.

Ticks are most usually found in heavily wooded areas and near stone walls where leaves from trees have accumulated. Adult ticks can also be found on top of long grass. If you live near areas such as these or are visiting, be especially careful. Use insect repellents containing DEET on children over two months of age when needed to prevent insect-related diseases, such as ticks, which can transmit Lyme disease, and mosquitoes, which can transmit West Nile Virus and other viruses.

Bee stings, while in most cases not as serious as Lyme disease, are another painful reality of summer. Unfortunately, children usually learn the hard way about avoiding bees and their hives. Help prevent your child from being stung by eliminating the use of fragrant shampoos or lotions. Similar to tick prevention, dress children in light-colored clothing. Check playground equipment and near windows for new hives. If you find one, keep your child away from the area until you can safely destroy it. Remind children not to drink directly out of soda cans as a bee could find its way into an open one without the child's realizing it. If you're having a picnic, clean up food as quickly as possible and keep children away from garbage cans where swarms of bees can gather.

After you've pulled the stinger out, wash the area with soap and water and place ice on it to prevent swelling; then rub some hydrocortisone on the infected area. You can also give your child an antihistamine, such as Children's Benadryl, to prevent the reaction from spreading. Watch your child for any sign of an allergic reaction, such as swelling, difficulty breathing, or nausea at which point you should call 911 immediately.

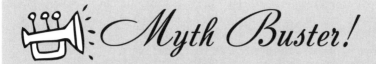

Removing a Bee Sting

Myth: If you are stung, never pull the stinger out with your fingers because this can send more venom into your body.

It is more important to get the stinger out of your child as soon as possible to reduce the risk of secondary infection. If additional venom is pumped in inadvertently, it will *not* increase the reaction.

Camping

I'll never forget when my cousin, the real out-doorsy type, told me that she was taking her three-month-old baby camping with her. This is something that she and her husband loved doing, and they were committed to just rolling their daughter right into their passion. Given that my idea of roughing it is staying in a motel room without a coffee maker, I found this incomprehensible. But there are other hearty souls like her out there, and yes, her daughter did survive, and they all seemed to have a great time.

If you're planning a camping trip with your baby understand that you'll need more provisions than you normally do. Even if you're nursing, you'll still need diapers, wipes, additional clothing, and other items. Bottle-feeding will obviously require much more planning. Premixed formula is much easier than powdered—just be sure to keep the cans cool until you use them. Don't forget that you'll need to boil the nipples before using them. If your baby is eating finger foods, think of bringing some that don't need to be refrigerated. In addition to the first aid items you normally take on a camping trip, remember a baby thermometer, acetaminophen or ibuprofen (but only if your child is over two years of age!), and diaper rash cream.

If your baby is able to sit up on her own, look for a sturdy baby carrier designed for hiking that also can include an attached backpack and sun shade. Look at some of the better sporting goods stores to find these. You can also find portable, inflatable cribs that will work nicely. As always, only place your baby on a firm surface to sleep, and never in a sleeping bag. Dress her appropriately as she can get hot in the carrier, and you want to watch for signs of dehydration.

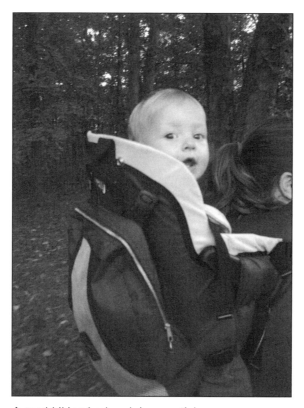

A good hiking backpack is essential.

You might want to nurse a bit more often and supplement with water, but only if she is over six months of age. Be sure to apply plenty of sunscreen, and if you're going hiking, keep her as shaded as possible. Remember however that neither sunscreen nor insect repellant should be applied to a baby under six months of age, even if they are "all-natural" or organic. Watch your child carefully to be sure she doesn't put any plants or leaves in her mouth that could be poisonous. State park Web sites often have poisonous plant listings that can be printed out and taken along for the trip.

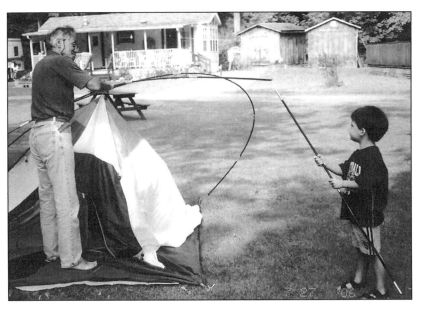

Camping is fun for the older kids as well.

Halloween Safety

Fall is undoubtedly my second most favorite season, and not just because the kids are finally going back to school. I love the clothes, the colors, and the crispness in the air. I'm not a big Halloween person, but my kids start planning their costumes by late August. I was so proud of myself that this year I actually made a homemade costume for my daughter (she was a cupcake). Whether you're big into Halloween or not, when it comes to kids, you need to put some safety measures in place to make sure that it stays fun for them.

The amount of candy that is consumed at Halloween is ridiculous. I've learned to purposely buy candy that I don't like so I'm not tempted to devour an entire bag. Carefully check out the candy your little ones get to avoid choking hazards. Children under five years of age should not be allowed to eat hard candy, caramels, popcorn, or items with nuts. All kids should be reminded to only eat candy that's unopened and in its original wrapper. Make sure that your children brush and rinse immediately after eating any Halloween candy. Consider handing out some safer alternatives such as stickers, temporary tattoos, pretzels, or fruit rollups.

When considering Halloween costumes, think about safety as well as cuteness! Try to create or select a costume in a lighter color, which is easier to see in the dark. Place a piece of reflective tape on both the front and back of the costume and also purchase a few glow bracelets or necklaces for your child to wear. For younger children, be sure there are no long strings near the collar of the costume, which could pose a strangulation hazard. Make sure that the costume is not too long, which could cause your child to trip. (One of the leading causes of accidents at Halloween is falls.)

Rather than wearing a mask, which might cause limited vision, try non-toxic paint and make-up to create a scary face. If possible, trick-or-treat in a community where the homes are close together and well lit or in a city, choose one or two apartment buildings in which you have friends. Only go to areas where there are sidewalks and street lamps. Stay away from homes and roads that are poorly lit. Remind your child never to enter a house, and always stay outside the door.

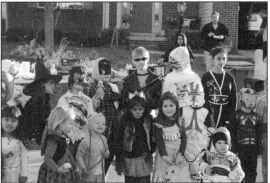 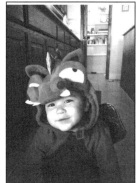

Halloween costumes can be cute *and* safe.

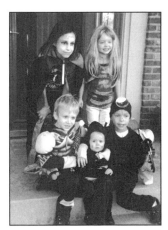 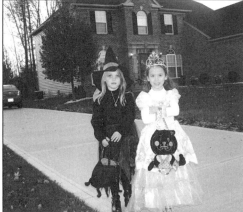

Birthday Parties

For a lot of parents, children's birthday parties have become major events. Many parents will spend extravagant amounts of money on their child's first birthday, only to have her sleep through the entire thing. What some parents might think is a perfect themed party could wind up being a disaster. I remember my son's first birthday. He loved Winnie the Pooh so I hired someone to come dressed up as Tigger. The guy was at least six feet tall and came bounding into the living room. My son took one look and started wailing. And that's when I learned that understated is sometimes better.

Party Details to Consider

No matter what sort of party you throw, you need to consider your guests as well as your own child. Time the party so that it's right after lunch when most kids are fed and contented. There's nothing worse than a bunch of cranky kids or hungry kids that you're trying to entertain. Make it very clear whether this is a drop-off party or not. Some parents will consider this free babysitting and leave their child with you for an additional hour after the party ends. If it is a drop-off party, make sure that you have enough adults to help you. As a rule of thumb, the number of guests should be limited to the age of the child. If it is a family party and you will be having children of different ages, be sure to have separate age appropriate activities that are equally safe for young and older children.

While it is a kid birthday party, try to serve at least one healthy food. A bunch of toddlers hopped up on too much sugar will make even the hardiest adult run for cover. Some foods to consider are drinkable yogurts, applesauce, or fruit cups. If the party is for children under five years of age, stay away from foods that are considered to be choking hazards, such as hot dogs, popcorn, whole grapes, raw carrots, and large chunks of cheese. Be sure that you are aware of any food allergies among your guests.

Consider your child's age and interests, as well as your budget when deciding on a theme and location. If you are having a pool party, find out from each parent their child's swimming ability prior to the party. If it's your pool, hire a lifeguard to be on duty during the party. When the children are in the pool, assign each guest a "buddy" and pair them up. Keep a cordless phone with you at the pool and be sure that you have recently taken a CPR course. If the party is at a public place such as a movie theater, mall, or restaurant, create fun, brightly colored t-shirts for all the guests so that it's easier to spot them in a crowd. Be sure that you've established a meeting place with the parents and get a cell phone number from each in case of an emergency.

If you have rented a "bounce house" or inflatable item, do not allow younger children and older children to be in it at the same time and limit the number of children on at any one time. This is also the case for a "pool of balls" where a younger child could lose his balance and get knocked over by an older friend or sibling. Purchase a piñata with pull strings rather than one that needs to be opened by hitting it with a stick.

Make sure that items in the party bags that guests will take home are age appropriate. For children under three, small bags of animal crackers, jars of bubbles, and small packages of crayons are a better alternative to candy.

Decorations and Balloons

One last consideration is decorations and balloons. Many people don't realize how dangerous latex balloons are. My kids used to think I was the meanest mom in the world because whenever they would come home from a birthday party with a balloon I'd pop it. Remarkably, balloons are the second leading cause of choking deaths for children. Accidents involving balloons tend to occur in two ways. Some children have sucked uninflated balloons into their mouths, often while attempting to inflate them. This can occur when a child who is blowing up the balloon inhales or takes a breath to prepare for the next blow and draws the balloon back into the mouth and throat. Some deaths may have resulted when children swallowed uninflated balloons they were sucking or chewing on. The Consumer Product Safety Commission knows of one case in which a child was chewing on an uninflated balloon when she fell from a swing. The child hit the ground and, in a reflex action, inhaled sharply. She suffocated on the balloon.

The second kind of accident involves balloon pieces. Children have drawn pieces of broken balloons that they were playing with into their throats. If a balloon breaks and is not discarded, for example, some children may continue to play with it, chewing on pieces of the balloon or attempting to stretch it across their mouths and suck or blow bubbles in it. These balloon pieces are easily sucked into the throat and lungs. Balloons mold to the throat and lungs and can completely block breathing.

Because of the danger of suffocation, the Consumer Products Safety Commission recommends that parents and guardians do not allow children under the age of eight to play with uninflated balloons without supervision. The CPSC does not believe that a completely inflated balloon presents a hazard to young children. If the balloon breaks, however, CPSC recommends that parents immediately collect the pieces of the broken balloon and dispose of them out of the reach of young children.

Don't put too much pressure on yourself to create the "perfect" birthday. It will be memorable, no matter what. Keep it simple and safe, and you all will have fun.

4th of July

For me, the 4th of July is the epitome of summer—barbecues, the beach, and warm summer nights. Naturally, a big part of this is the fireworks. They're romantic, nostalgic, and exciting all at the same time. For years, my kids didn't share this view. I remember many holidays being forced to watch the Macy's fireworks on TV because my kids were completely freaked out by the noise. It's understandable, but I was happy when they all got over it, and we were able to enjoy the town fireworks together as a family.

Needless to say, there are some inherent dangers built in to this holiday. In 2007, approximately 7,000 people were treated in emergency rooms for fireworks-related injuries and half of these were children under the age of 15. I remember being at a party one year and watching a dad shoot off fireworks with a bunch of kids nearby. It absolutely made me cringe.

But it's not just fireworks. Sparklers caused half of the injuries to children under the age of five. The same parents who wouldn't ever allow their children to go near matches for some reason see no problem with them holding sparklers at 4th of July. What they probably don't realize is that sparklers can get as hot as 1,000 degrees! While sparklers are fun, I've found that my kids enjoy glow-in-the-dark necklaces just as much.

There are a few safety precautions to consider when going to a professional fireworks display:

* It will be dark when the show starts, so make sure if your kids are wandering around that they are back with you before dark. Choose a spot that will be easy to leave when the fireworks end.

* Put a piece of reflective tape on the back of their clothes to help keep track of them as you're leaving and always bring two flashlights with you (in case the batteries run out on one). Watch for broken glass and other hazards that you might trip on as you leave.

* Be sure your kids know your cell phone number and address in case they get lost on the way out.

* If your kids are going to a fireworks show with a friend, give the parents a recent photo of your child and memorize what clothes they were wearing so that you can easily describe them to officials.

There will be so many special moments in your child's life and some of the best are the impromptu ones. Those times that aren't planned and choreographed but simply evolve. Whether we're trying to re-create memories from our childhood or create ones that we never had the opportunity to experience, we put terrible pressure on ourselves to make every holiday, celebration, and event perfect. At the end of the day, our kids love nothing better than relaxing and laughing with us.

Conclusion

I honestly never thought I'd write a book. But then again, there are so many things in life that we think we'll never do until we're thrown into a situation. My journey and mission as The Safety Mom is completely due to the greatest tragedy in my life—the death of my son Connor. I wish with all of my heart it wouldn't have happened, and even though I know that SIDS is unpreventable, there's somewhere in the back of my mind that I still wonder if there's something I could have done differently. But he gave me the greatest gifts of my life—the courage to do a job that inspires me every day, empathy to realize that everyone has "a story," and the appreciation of living every day with my family.

As parents, we question our decisions every day, and I doubt that ever ends. But the reality is that none of us is perfect, as much as we might try. It's always going to be trial and error, and we just need to know in our hearts that we're doing the absolute best we can for our kids. Learn as much as you can, trust in your heart, and lead with a little faith.

Diaper Bag Checklist

Diapering
- ❏ Extra diapers, at least 6 or 7
- ❏ Wipes
- ❏ Diaper rash cream
- ❏ A washable mat for diaper changing
- ❏ Plastic diaper bags for dirty diapers

Feeding
- ❏ Extra formula and bottles (if you are not nursing) and sippy cups
- ❏ Burping cloths
- ❏ Two bottles of water, one for you and one for formula
- ❏ If baby is eating solids, snacks
- ❏ Baby food in non-breakable jar
- ❏ Utensils
- ❏ Plastic bag to throw away garbage

Soothing & Comfort
- ❏ Two lightweight blankets
- ❏ Two baby toys
- ❏ Teething ring
- ❏ Stuffed animal
- ❏ Crayons or toys
- ❏ Extra pacifier

First Aid
- ❏ Nasal syringe
- ❏ Thermometer
- ❏ Saline spray
- ❏ Band-Aids/first aid ointment
- ❏ Antihistamine
- ❏ Fever reducer
- ❏ Sun screen
- ❏ Bug repellent
- ❏ Tissues

Just in Case
- ❏ Extra undershirt and socks
- ❏ Plastic bag for soiled clothing
- ❏ Emergency phone list, including poison control, pediatrician, secondary emergency contact, medical insurance information, and list of any medical issues your baby might have

Just for Mom
- ❏ Extra shirt
- ❏ Extra nursing pad
- ❏ Small pack with cell phone, keys, money, credit card, ID, and lip gloss

Honey, I Lost the Baby in the Produce Aisle!

Nanny Questionnaire

Name of Applicant: _____

Home Phone Number: _____

Cell Phone Number: _____

Home Address: _____

Emergency Contact: _____

1. What is your educational background?
   _____

2. Do you have any formal early childhood development education or training?
   _____

3. How long have you been a nanny?
   _____

4. During the above time period, how many families did you work for on a full-_
   time basis?
   _____

5. How many on a part-time basis?
   _____

6. Have you done live-in or live-out?
   _____

7. How long were you in your last position?
   _____

8. Why did you leave your last position?
   _____

9. What did you like the most/least about your last family?
   _____

10. What were the ages of the children you were responsible for?
    _____

11. What do children like best about you?
    _____

12. Did you drive the children?
    _____

13. Whose car did you drive?
    _____

14. Did you cook for the children? Give a sample menu for each meal of the day.
    _____

15. Name a few of the snacks you would normally allow a child.
    _____

16. Did you bathe the children?
    _____

17. Detail the nighttime bathing routine.
    _____

18. How did you handle bathroom safety?

19. What traits do you possess that you feel qualify you to take care of children?

20. Have you ever been arrested?

21. Do you smoke?

22. Are you CPR certified?

23. When was the last time you took a CPR refresher course?

24. Have you ever taken a First Aid course?

25. List a few activities you would do with the children to stimulate learning.

26. How would you handle a situation of one child biting another?

27. What is the most important responsibility of a nanny?

28. Have you ever had to handle an emergency situation? Explain.

29. Describe your ideal family to work for.

30. How do you comfort a scared or hurt child?

31. How do you discipline a child?

32. How do you reward a child?

33. How do you handle stress?

34. What type of situation causes you stress?

35. List three references. Include the following information: Name, address, length of employment, and the number and ages of the children.

Au Pair Questionnaire

Name of Applicant: _____

Home Phone Number: _____

Cell Phone Number: _____

Home Address: _____

Emergency Contact: _____

1. Is this your first time living outside of your home country?
   _____

2. How do you think you will adjust to living in another country?
   _____

3. Have you previously done any international traveling?
   _____

4. Do you think you can live away from your family and friends?
   _____

5. Have you ever been an au pair before?
   _____

6. Why do you want to be an au pair?
   _____

7. How well do you comprehend the English language?
   _____

8. Where did you learn to speak English?
   _____

9. Did you grow up in a large city or a rural area?
   _____

10. How long have you been driving and how much driving do you do?
    _____

11. Do you have a U.S. drivers license?
    _____

12. How would you spend your weekends?
    _____

13. How do you think this experience will change you as a person?

14. What are your plans after your au pair experience?

15. Provide three references with the following information: name, phone number and address, length of employment, number and ages of children.

Index

A

abduction, 134
accredited day care center, 173
ACNM (American College of Nurse-Midwives), 6
activity center, 23–25
adhesive-mount cabinet lock, 62
ADT Home Pulse Monitoring system, 171
ADT Home Security System, 43
airport security, 140–141
alarm
    carbon monoxide (CO), 42–43
    smoke, 41
    stick-on, 151
allergies, 129–130
American College of Nurse-Midwives (ACNM), 6
America's Most Wanted (John Walsh), 188
AmSafe Aviation CARES harness, 142
amusement park, 127–128
anchors, 55
appliances, kitchen, 81–83
Arm's Reach co-sleeper, 11
Asperger's Syndrome, 99
asthma, 195
au pair
    ages of, 163
    benefits of, 164
    challenges of using, 166–168
    exchange visitor visa, 165
    language barriers, 167
    resources, 165
    state department guidelines, 165–166

autism
    Centers of Disease Control statistics, 98
    diagnosis, 98
    divorce and, 101
    ID bracelet, 104
    lead poison linked to, 109–110
    medical problems related to, 100
    motion detectors for children with, 103–104
    parental feeling of guilt, 102
    support for, 101–103
    symptoms, 99–100
Autism Speaks Web site, 102
AutoLock pressure gate (Cardinal), 47
automatic door closer, 68

B

Baby Care Centers (theme park), 157
"baby-blues," 39–40
BabyGo High Chair (Evenflo), 149
babyproofer, 46
babysitter
    au pairs, 164–168
    background check, 178
    childcare debate, 164
    day care centers, 172–175
    family day care, 176–177
    finding, 177–178
    First Aid certified, 178
    grandparent as, 148–151
    nannies, 168–172
    reviewing evacuation plan with, 178
    working parents and, 162–163

BabySuite Select play yard (Evenflo), 20

Back To Sleep campaign, 148

back *versus* **tummy sleeping,** 38–39

Baker, Virginia Graeme, 126

background check, babysitter, 178

back-over accidents, 92

backpack, 198–199

balloons, 203

baluster mounting kit, 51

baseboard, 55

bath toy, 27

bath tub, 25–26, 87

bath tub ring, 26

bathroom safety, 86–87

batteries, 186

beach safety, 122–126

bedbug infestation, 152–153

bee sting, 197–198

Benadryl, 122, 197

benzyl benzoate, 108

bicycle, 115–117

bi-fold locks, 71–72

birth certificate, 136, 142

birthday party, 202–203

birthing center, 6

bisphenol-A (BPA), 106–107

blanket, 13

Boarding Verification Document, 142

bolt
    pocket door, 73
    surface, 69
    toggle, 54–55

booster seat
    and high chair combination, 21–22
    for travel, 149

bottle feeding on plane, 145

bounce house, 203

bouncy seat, 23–25

BPA (bisphenol-A), 106–107

brain injury, 116

buddy system, 202

BurglaBar flip lock, 58–60

bullying, 117–118

C

cabinet lock. *See* drawer/cabinet lock

camera, nanny cam, 170–171

camping safety, 198–199

candy, 200

car seat
    convertible, 16
    five-point harness system, 18
    infant, 14
    LATCH (Lower Anchors and Tethers for Children) system, 13
    mirror for, 18
    on plane, 141–144
    positioning and installation, 17–18
    recliner settings, 16
    selection considerations, 13
    taxi regulation, 18–19
    travel system, 15
    used, 11

carbon monoxide (CO), 42–43

Cardinal
    AutoLock pressure gate, 47
    Stairway Special Safety gate, 47
    VersaGate, 49

cardiopulmonary resuscitation (CPR), 124, 178

caregiver. *See* babysitter

carnivals, 127–128

Centers of Disease Control, 98

cerebral palsy, 104–105

Certified Midwife (CM), 6

Certified Nurse-Widwife (CNM), 6

Certified Professional Midwife (CPM), 6

chain door guards, 69

chemical toxins, 106–107

child abduction, 134

child restraint system (CRS), 141–143

Childhood Disintegrative Disorder, 99

"Children at Play" signs, 103

child-tracking device/locator, 156

choking hazard, 184

Christmas
children's expectations of, 180–182
decorations, 184
lights, 182
ornament, 182
parties, 184–185
pressure during, 180–182
trees, 182–183
clean air, 108
cleaning products, 108–109
clothing
camping, 198
outside play, 112
theme park, 157
winter safety, 190–191
CO (carbon monoxide), 42–43
"Code Adam" (Adam Walsh), 188–189
Coffee Klatch Web site, 103
cold germs, 112
condos, 155
Consumer Product Safety Commission (CPSC)
balloon suffocation, 203
bicycle helmet safety, 116
high chair accidents, 21
as information source, 10
Lyme disease, 195
playground safety guidelines, 120
recalls, 10
shopping cart injuries, 131
topple-over accident statistics, 74
trampoline injury, 193–194
convertible car seat, 16
cooking with kids, 84–85, 185
cord blood banking, 2–4
cord covers, 89
cord, window blind, 61–62
co-sleeping, 11
costumes, 200–201
CPM (Certified Professional Midwife), 6
CPR (cardiopulmonary resuscitation), 124, 178

CPSC. *See* Consumer Product Safety Commission
Cresci Window Wedge, 58
crib
bumper, 13
drop-side, 11
mattress, 13
old, 149
pillow and blankets in, 13
tent, 33
used, 11
CRS (child restraint system), 141–143
cruises, 156
C-section, 5–6

D

day care centers
benefits of, 172
family day care, 176–177
frequent visits to, 175
hours of operation, 172
researching, 173–175
Decora outlet cover, 87–88
decoration
birthday party, 203
Christmas, 184
dehydration, 195
depression, postpartum, 39–40
diaper bag accessories, 113–115
diaper changing, 144–145
disaster preparedness kit, 42
discipline, day care center, 174
Disney, 158
divorce and autism, 101
dogs, 30–33
DONA International Web site, 6
door
drawer/cabinet lock, 65–66
lock installation
automatic door closer, 68
bi-fold locks, 71–72
chain door guards, 69
flip locks, 69

front-mount door closer, 69
importance of, 67
pocket door bolts, 73
shutter bars, 72
surface bolts, 69
top-of-door lock, 70–71
doula, 6
down time, 132
drain, pool, 126
drawer/cabinet lock
flush drawer, 63
installation
door lock, 65
flush frame door lock, 65
flush frame drawer lock, 64–65
interior hardware-mounted cabinet lock, 63–64
one-piece lock, 65–66
Wonder Latch, 66–67
overlay drawer, 63
types of, 62
driveway, 92
drop-side crib, 11
drowning prevention, 124–125, 194–195
Dutch Wonderland, 158

E

eating disorder, 100
electrical cords, 73–74
elevator safety, 153
emergency
bicycle-related injury, 116
escape ladder, 41
evacuation plan, 34, 40–42
fire drill, 41
fireworks injury, 204
environmental toxins, 106–109
escalators, 189–190
escape ladder, 41
EuroTrek Travel System (Evenflo), 15

evacuation plan
guidelines, 40–42
for hotel and resort, 154–155
reviewing with babysitter, 178
Evenflo
BabyGo High Chair, 149
BabySuite Select play yard, 20
EuroTrek Travel System, 15
ExerSaucer Jump & Learn Active Learning Center, 24
Maestro convertible car seat, 16
Secure System infant car seat, 14
Symphony car set, 17
exercise room, 90
ExerSaucer Jump & Learn Active Learning Center (Evenflo), 24
exterior cabinet lock, 62

F

4th of July, 204
Facebook, 134
fall-related injury, 57
"family bed," 11
family day care, 176–177
fence, pool, 93–94, 151
fire
Christmas tree, 183
reality of, 152
fire drill, 41
fire extinguisher, 40–41
fire hazards, kitchen, 84
fireworks, 204
First Aid certified babysitter, 178
first aid kit
for camping, 198
items needed in, 42
playground, 122
First Alert Carbon Monoxide Detector, 42
First Candle/SIDS Alliance, 38
five-point harness system, 18
flight. *See* plane preparation and safety
flip lock, 69

flush drawer, 63
food
    allergy, 129–130
    birthday party, 202
    in day care centers, 174
    at family day cares, 177
    organic, 109
    pesticides used in, 109
food court germs, 190
front-mount door closer, 69
frostbite and frost nip, 192
furniture
    home office, 89
    used, 11–12
furniture strapping and bracing
    installation
    bracing, 75–76
    furniture straps, 74–75
    L-bracket install, 75–76
    wood rail install, 75

G

garage, 91
garbage cans, 80
gardening tools, 90
gastrointestinal (GI) problems, 100
gate
    extensions, 51
    hardware-mounted, 47–48, 52–53
    hearth, 50
    installation
        baseboard considerations, 55
        in brick or cement wall, 55
        hardware-mounted, 52–53
        materials needed, 51
        newel post kit, 56
        stairway installs, 53
        toggle bolt, 54–55
    pressure-mounted, 49
    pressure-mounted walk-through,
        48–49
    retractable, 50
    sectional, 49–50, 56–57

spiral staircase, 56
types, 47
wood *versus* metal, 50
germs
    from common cold, 112
    food court, 190
    spread of, 35
GFI (ground fault interruption)
    switch, 87
GI (gastrointestinal) problems, 100
grandparent babysitting, 148–151
grease fire, 84–85
grills, 90, 194
ground covering, playground, 121
ground fault interruption (GFI)
    switch, 87
Guardian Angel Web site, 59
gym, 90

H

Halloween safety, 200–201
halogen lamps, 89
Hanukkah, 180
    menorahs, 184
hand-me-downs, 11–12
hand washing, 35, 84
hardware-mounted gate, 47–48,
    52–53
harness system, 142–143
head injury, 191
hearing test, 8
hearth gate, 50
helmet
    bicycle, 116
    ski, 191–192
high chair, 21–22, 149
hiking backpack, 198–199
hives, 197
holiday and special occasions
    birthday party, 202–203
    camping, 198–199
    Christmas and Hanukkah, 180–190
    4th of July, 204

Halloween, 200–201
holiday cooking, 185
lost children, 188–189
shopping safety, 187–188
summer safety, 193–197
toys, 186
winter safety, 190–192
home gym, 90
home office, 88–89
hook-on high chair, 22
hot tub, 93–94, 151
hotel and resort
bedbug infestation, 152–153
elevator safety, 153
evacuation planning, 154–155
fitness area, 155
hazards, 153–154
kid friendly, 152
orienting children to, 153
pools, 155
household cleaners, 108–109
hydration, 134, 195
hyper-sensitivity, 100
hypo-sensitivity, 100

I

ice-skating, 192
ID bracelet, 104
infant car seat, 14
infant co-sleeper, 11
inspection report, day care center, 173
installation
BurglaBars, 60
cord cleats, 62
door lock
bi-fold locks, 71–72
chain door guards, 69
flip locks, 69
front-mount door closer, 69
importance of, 68
pocket door bolts, 73
shutter bars, 72

surface bolts, 69
top-of-door lock, 70–71
drawer/cabinet lock
door lock, 65
flush frame door clock, 65
flush frame drawer lock, 64–65
interior hardware-mounted
cabinet lock, 63–64
one-piece lock, 65–66
Wonder Latch, 66–67
furniture strapping and bracing
bracing, 75–76
L-bracket install, 75–76
straps, 74–75
wood rail install, 75
gate
baseboard considerations, 55
in brick or cement wall, 55
hardware-mounted, 52–53
materials needed, 51
newel post kit, 56
stairway installs, 53–54
toggle bolt, 54–55
looped blind cords, 62
sliding window locks, 60
wedge locks and window stops, 60
window guards, 61
Window Wedge, 59
International Association for Child Safety Web site, 46
interview with nanny, 169–170

J

JPMA (Juvenile Products Manufacturers Association), 10

K

KidCo
Adhesive/Hardware-mount lock, 62
toilet lock, 86
kitchen safety
appliances, 81–83
cooking with kids, 84–85

fire hazards, 84
garbage cans, 80
hot grease, 84–85
oven locks, 84
refrigerator lock, 80
safe area setup, 79–80
stove guards and shields, 81–83
washers and dryers, 81
water coolers, 80

L

lamps, 89
language barriers, au pair, 167
LATCH (Lower Anchors and Tethers for Children) system, 13
lawn mower, 92
L-bracket, 75–76
lead, 109–110
learning disability, 96
license
family day care, 176
public day care center, 173
life vest, 124–125
lights, Christmas tree, 182
Looking Glass Window Guard Web site, 59
looped blind chords, 62
lost children, 188–189
Lower Anchors and Tethers for Children (LATCH) system, 13
Lyme disease, 195–197

M

Maestro convertible car seat (Evenflo), 16
Magic Kingdom, 158
magnetic cabinet lock, 62
MANA (Midwives Alliance of North America), 6
mattress, 13
Measles, Mumps, Rubella (MMR) vaccine, 102

media room, 90
medication
Benadryl, 122, 197
Neosporin, 122
Pitocin, 5
medicine cabinet lock, 87
menorahs, 184
metabolic disorder, 7–8
metal *versus* **wood gate,** 50
midwife, 4–6
Midwives Alliance of North America (MANA), 6
miscarriage, 7
MMR (Measles, Mumps, Rubella) vaccine, 102
motion detectors, 103–104
myth
bee sting, 198
cold germs, 112
cord blood banking, 4
day care benefits, 172
divorce and autism, 101
eating and drowning, 126
germs and disease-causing organisms, 86
germs and planes, 145
short fall, 57
tummy *versus* back sleeping, 39

N

NAEYC (National Association for the Education of Young Children), 173
NAFCC (National Association for Family Child Care), 173
nannies
benefits of, 169
cost of, 169
detailing a list of expectations for, 171–172
interviewing, 169–170
nanny cam, 170–171

nap area
  in day care center, 174
  at family day care, 177
National Association for the Education of Young Children (NAEYC), 173
National Association for Family Child Care (NAFCC), 173
National Highway Traffic Safety Administration, 17
National Newborn Screening & Genetics Resource Center Web site, 8
natural child birth, 4–6
natural disasters and travel warnings, 138–139
Neosporin, 122
newborn screening test, 7–8
newel post kit, 56
no hole mounting kit, 51–52
NPPS (National Program for Playground Safety) Playground Report Card, 120

O
organic food, 109
ornament, Christmas tree, 182
outdoor play area, 92
outdoor terrace railing, 90
outlet cover, 87–88, 150–151
outside play
  amusement parks and carnivals, 127–128
  child abductions, 134
  clothing for, 112
  drowning prevention, 124–126
  gear needed for, 113–115
  playground equipment, 117–122
  pools and beaches, 122–123
  protection from sun, 112
  riding toy safety, 115–117
  sports, 132–133
oven lock, 84
overlay drawer, 63

P
packing
  for flight, 139–140
  for vacation, 137–138
paint, lead, 109–110
parenthood, 29
parties, 184–185
passports, 136–137
PDD (Pervasive Developmental Disorder), 99
PDD-NOS (Pervasive Developmental Disorder-Not Specific), 99
peanut butter, 130
Pervasive Developmental Disorder-Not Specific (PDD-NOS), 99
Pervasive Developmental Disorder (PDD), 99
pesticides, 109
pets, 30–33, 81, 150–151
phthalates, 106–107
Pica, 100
pick pocketing, 138
Pitocin, 5
plane preparation and safety
  airport security, 140–141
  Boarding Verification Document, 142
  bottle feeding on plane, 145
  car seat and child restraints, 141–144
  diaper changing on plane, 144–145
  packing, 139–140
  vest and harness system, 142–143
plastic consumer products, 106
play dates, 128–131
play yard, 20–21, 118–121
playground
  bullying on, 117
  CPSC safety guidelines, 120
  at day care center, 174
  first aid kit, 122
  ground covering, 121
  interaction with other children, 118
  old equipment, 121
Playground Report Card (NPPS), 120
Playground Safety Web site, 120

pocket door bolts, 73
Poison Control, 78
pool
  drain, 126
  drowning prevention, 124–125,
    194–195
  fence around, 93–94, 151
  hotel and resort, 155
porch and patio, 90–91
postpartum depression, 39–40
power tools, 91
pregnancy
  midwife and doula roles and respon-
    sibilities during, 4–6
  stillbirth and miscarriage, 7
premature birth, 105
pressure-mounted gate, 49
pressure-mounted walk-through
  gate, 48–49
product reviews, 10

R
recalls
  automatic email alert, 10
  drop-side crib, 11
  toy, 186
refrigerator lock, 80
respiratory syncytial virus (RSV),
  35–36
retractable gate, 50
Rett Syndrome, 99
ride-on toys, 115–117
road trips, 145–146
Roman Shades, 61
room temperature, 38
RSV (respiratory syncytial virus),
  35–36

S
Safety Certification Seal (JPMA), 10
Safety Mom Solutions Web site, 46
safety zone area, 34–35

sandbox, 92
scanner, airport security, 140–141
Sea World, 158
seatbelt, 142
secondhand smoke, 38
sectional gate, 49–50, 56–57
Secure System infant car seat
  (Evenflo), 14
Sensory Integration Disorder, 100
sex offenders, 134
sheets, 13
Shields, Brooke, 39
shopping cart injury, 131–132
shopping safety, 187–190
short fall, 57
shutter bars, 72
siblings
  help from, 34
  jealousy among, 33
SIDS (Sudden Infant Death
  Syndrome), 36–38
ski resorts, 159–160
sledding, 191
sleep problems, 100
slip-resistant mat
  bath tub, 87
  home office, 89
smoke alarm, 41, 174
Snooze Sack, 13
Snooze Wrap, 13
snow, winter safety, 190–191
snowboarding, 191–192
space heater, 41
special education needs, 96–97
special needs children. See autism;
  cerebral palsy
speech pathology, 96
spiral staircase gate, 56
sports
  overscheduled, 132–133
  parent peer pressure, 134
  winter safety, 191–192
spring latch, 62

stairway gate installation, 53–54
Stairway Special Safety gate
    (Cardinal), 47
state department guidelines, au
    pair, 165–166
stay-at-home parents, 162–163
stem cell, cord blood, 4
stick-on alarm, 151
stillbirth, 7
stove guards and shields, 81–83
strangulation hazards
    electrical cord, 73
    window blind cords, 61
stroller, 15
Sudden Infant Death Syndrome
    (SIDS), 36–38
summer safety
    camping, 198–199
    dehydration, 195
    drowning, 194–195
    equipment checking, 193
    grilling, 194
    Lyme disease and bee stings, 195–197
    sunscreen, 194
    trampolines, 193–194
sunscreen, 112, 194, 199
support for autism, 101–103
surf warning, 127
surface bolts, 69
swim lessons, 124
swing set, 92
swivel lock, 62
Symphony car seat (Evenflo), 17

T

tandem mass spectrometry, 8
tannic acid, 108
tapcon, 55
taxi
    accidents in, 19
    and car seat regulation, 18–19
tent, crib, 33

terrace and outdoor deck, 90
theft, 138
theme parks, 156–158
ticks, 197
toggle bolt, 54–55
toilet lock, 86
top-of-door lock, 70–71
Tot-Locks, 62
toxins, 106–109
toys
    age appropriate, 186
    bath, 27
    Christmas, 186
    in day care centers, 174
    hazardous, 186
    recalls, 186
trampoline, 122, 193–194
travel
    booster seat, 149
    condos, 155
    cruises, 156
    high chair for, 149
    hotel and resorts, 152–155
    natural disasters and travel warnings,
        138–139
    packing for, 137–138
    passports, 136–137
    plane and flight preparation, 139–145
    road trips, 145–146
    ski resorts, 159–160
    theme parks, 156–158
    visas, 136
travel system, 15. See also car seat
tricycle, 115–117
tummy versus back sleeping, 38–39
Tyson, Mike, 90

U

used car seat, 11
used crib, 11
used furniture and products, 11–12

V

vacation. *See* travel
vaccination, 102, 136
ventilation, 108
VersaGate (Cardinal), 49
vinyl flooring, 107
Virginia Graeme Baker Pool & Spa Safety Act, 126
visas, 136

W

Wakefield, Andrew, 102
Walsh, Adam, 188–189
Walsh, John, 188
washers and dryers, 81
water coolers, 80
Web site
  American College of Nurse-Midwives (ACNM), 6
  Autism Speaks, 102
  Coffee Klatch, 103
  DONA International, 6
  First Candle/SIDS Alliance, 38
  Guardian Angel, 59
  International Association for Child Safety, 46
  Looking Glass Window Guard, 59

  Midwives Alliance of North America (MANA), 6
  National Newborn Screening & Genetics Resource Center, 8
  Playground Safety, 120
  Safety Mom Solutions, 46
window
  BurglaBar flip lock, 58–60
  falls from, 57
  guards, 61
  Roman Shades, 61
  sliding window locks, 60
  types, 57
  wedge locks and window stops, 60
  window blind cords, 61–62
  Window Wedge, 58–59
winter safety, 190–192
wires, home office, 89
Wonder Latch, 62, 66–67
wood rails
  furniture bracing installation, 75
  gate installation, 51
wood *versus* metal gate, 50
working parents, 162–163

Y

Yates, Andrea, 39

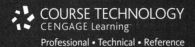
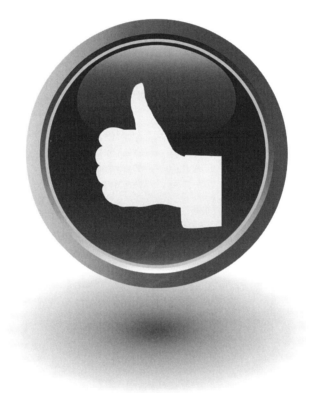

Babyproofing Shopping List

Product	Qty
Electrical Safety	
Decora Outlet Covers	_____
Standard Outlet Covers	_____
Cord Plug Cover	_____
Power Strip Cover	_____

Cabinet Safety

Door Locks	_____
Drawer Locks	_____

Window Safety

Window Wedges	_____
Cord Cleats	_____

Door Safety

Doorknob Cover	_____
Surface Bolts	_____
Door Stop (one piece)	_____

Bathroom Safety

Faucet Cover	_____
Toilet Lock	_____
Anti-Slip Bathtub Mat	_____
Anti-Slip Floor Mat	_____

Safety Gate

Location: _____
Type: _____
Width: _____

Safety Gate

Location: _____
Type: _____
Width: _____

Safety Gate

Location: _____
Type: _____
Width: _____

Safety Gate

Location: _____
Type: _____
Width: _____

Day Care Questionnaire

Name of Day Care Center: _____

Center Address: _____

Center Phone Number: _____

Contact Name: _____

General Business

_____ 1. How long has this facility been in business?

_____ 2. Do you have a current valid license and can you provide a copy?

_____ 3. Have you ever had a charge brought against you?

_____ 4. What are the hours of operation?

_____ 5. Are there late pick-up fees? If so, what are they?

_____ 6. How do you communicate with parents (via phone, email, etc.)?

_____ 7. What supplies do I need to send with my child and what does your facility provide?

_____ 8. Do you have parent references whom I can speak with?

Staffing

_____ 1. Have background checks been completed on all staff members?

_____ 2. Have all teachers and potential substitutes been fingerprinted? And have criminal and child abuse background checks been conducted?

_____ 3. What is the educational and experience level of the staff?

_____ 4. What is the staff-to-child ratio?

_____ 5. Is your staff required to have CPR and First Aid certification? Are they required to take refresher courses on a regular and consistent basis?

Safe Sleep Practices

_____ 1. Do you follow SIDS risk-reduction guidelines?

_____ 2. Do all infants sleep on their backs?

_____ 3. Do all cribs have firm mattresses?

_____ 4. Are the cribs free of loose blankets and stuffed animals?

Emergency & Fire Procedures

_____ 1. What happens in an emergency?

_____ 2. What pediatrician and hospital are you affiliated with?

_____ 3. Do you have an on-site nurse?

_____ 4. Do you have an adequate stock of first aid products?

_____ 5. Do you have a fire escape plan posted? Are the exits prominently displayed?

_____ 6. Are fire drills conducted on a regular basis?

_____ 7. What is the protocol if the building needs to be evacuated during the day?

_____ 8. Where are the children taken?

Outdoor Play Safety

_____ 1. Is the fence at least four feet in height and surrounding the entire perimeter?

_____ 2. Do you have at least 12 inches of wood chips, mulch, sand or pea gravel, or mats made of safety tested rubber or rubber-like material in the play area?

_____ 3. Is there a separate area for the infants to play away from the older children?

_____ 4. What are the temperature guidelines for outdoor play?

Indoor Play Safety

_____ 1. Do the smaller children have access to small toys, which are appropriate only for the older children?

_____ 2. Is the play area free of sharp, hard edges?

_____ 3. Do the play area surfaces and toys appear clean? How often are they cleaned?

_____ 4. What types of cleaning products are used for maintenance?

_____ 5. Do you have an outside cleaning company that maintains the facility?

Food Safety

_____ 1. What sort of food is being served at lunchtime and snacks?

_____ 2. What are the procedures regarding food allergies?

_____ 3. What rules are in place to avoid potential choking hazards?

_____ 4. How do you clean dishes, pots, and utensils (dishwasher, hand, etc.)?

Babyproofing

_____ 1. Are all electrical outlets not in use covered?

_____ 2. Are outdoor areas near water fenced and off limits?

_____ 3. Are all staircases gated?

_____ 4. Are refrigerators, ovens, and dishwashers locked?

_____ 5. Are window blind cords tied up and out of reach?

_____ 6. Are garages, basements, and laundry rooms kept locked at all times?

_____ 7. Is heavy furniture that could potentially topple over bolted to the wall?

_____ 8. Are all cleaning fluids and other toxic chemicals locked away and out of reach at all times?

_____ 9. Are cabinets that children shouldn't have access to installed with safety locks?

_____ 10. Are the windows gated or do they have locks that allow them to open only four inches?

_____ 11. Are the slats on cribs no more than 2 3/8" apart?

_____ 12. Are you using drop-side cribs?

Security

_____ 1. Are all doors to the facility locked from the inside at all times?

_____ 2. If a family day care setting, what is the policy regarding visitors at the home during operational hours? Is there a guarantee that any "personal" visitors to the home do not have a criminal background?

_____ 3. Are parents allowed to drop in and pay surprise visits at any time?